97 Organic Juice and Meal Recipes For People Who Suffer From Heart Disease:

Give Your Heart the Tools It Needs to Get Stronger!

By

Joe Correa CSN

COPYRIGHT

ACKNOWLEDGEMENTS

This book is dedicated to my friends and family that have had mild or serious illnesses so that you may find a solution and make the necessary changes in your life.

97 Organic Juice and Meal Recipes For People Who Suffer From Heart Disease:

Give Your Heart the Tools It Needs to Get Stronger!

By

Joe Correa CSN

CONTENTS

ABOUT THE AUTHOR

After years of Research, I honestly believe in the positive effects that proper nutrition can have over the body and mind. My knowledge and experience has helped me live healthier throughout the years and which I have shared with family and friends. The more you know about eating and drinking healthier, the sooner you will want to change your life and eating habits.

Nutrition is a key part in the process of being healthy and living longer so get started today. The first step is the most important and the most significant.

INTRODUCTION

97 Organic Juice and Meal Recipes For People Who Suffer From Heart Disease: Give Your Heart the Tools It Needs to Get Stronger!

By Joe Correa CSN

Heart disease is the number one cause of death in the world. A wide range of conditions that affect the heart can become a serious problem for middle-aged as well as older people. Once the disease is diagnosed, it lasts for life which is why your doctor will advise some medications and lifestyle changes. This part is crucial in keeping the condition under control. On the contrary, heart disease will get worse over time.

Heart disease is a serious problem all over the world. The lack of exercise, an inadequate diet, and other unhealthy habits can negatively affect the cardiovascular system. Making a consistent change to your diet is the first and most important step to having a stronger heart and a longer life.

Fortunately, changing lifestyle choices, a healthy diet, and moderate exercise can reduce the risk of getting heart disease, or at least, control the existing condition.

A diet low in saturated fat and trans fats is essential. Eating fruits and vegetables, fiber rich foods, whole grains and fish are delicious options. These recipes will help you enjoy delicious meals and keep you on the right track towards a healthy heart.

This book will provide you with a collection of delicious and tasty juice and meal recipes that will help you clean your body and improve your health. These juices are based on a variety of fresh fruits and vegetables that are proven to help clean blood vessels and ease the everyday functions of your heart.

Start with one recipe and then try them all. Make your heart stronger one day at a time with these great recipes!

97 ORGANIC JUICE AND MEAL RECIPES FOR PEOPLE WHO SUFFER FROM HEART DISEASE: GIVE YOUR HEART THE TOOLS IT NEEDS TO GET STRONGER!

MEALS

1.   Roasted Vegetable Penne

With a variety of vegetables, this simple pasta dish is packed with essential amino acids, vitamins, minerals, and flavor! This pasta dish is sure to boost heart function.

Ingredients:

- 10 ounces whole grain Penne
- 1 cup cherry or grape tomatoes, halved
- 1 cup asparagus, chopped
- 1 red bell pepper, sliced
- 1 purple onion, sliced
- 1 clove garlic, minced
- 1/2 tablespoon olive oil

- 1 tablespoon basil pesto

How to Prepare:

Preheat oven to 400 degrees.

Place asparagus, halved tomatoes, garlic red pepper, and onion in an oven-safe skillet or baking sheet. Drizzle with olive oil and roast for about 15 minutes, until vegetables have browned in places and asparagus is tender. Remove from the oven.

Toss pesto and pasta together, add vegetables and toss to combine.

Nutritional Information:

Total calories: 315

Vitamins: Vitamin A 210 µg, Vitamin B6 0.5mg, Vitamin B12 0.9 µg, Vitamin K 98µg

Minerals: Calcium 444mg, Potassium 1050mg, Riboflavin 0.5mg, Niacin 6mg

Sugars: 15g

2.   One Dish Chicken and Summer Vegetables

Packed with magnesium and other essential vitamins and minerals, this zucchini helps with blood flow and healthy cardio vascular activity. The body uses magnesium in over 300 different ways, many of which are in the heart.

Ingredients

- 4 boneless and skinless chicken breasts
- 1 medium zucchini, sliced into quarters
- 1 yellow squash, sliced into quarters
- 1 cup small tomatoes, halved
- 1/2 cup shredded parmesan cheese
- 2 tablespoons extra-virgin olive oil
- 1 teaspoon dried thyme
- 2 cloves garlic, sliced

How to prepare:

Preheat oven to 350 degrees.

Toss zucchini, squash, garlic, and some small tomatoes, and thyme in olive oil and spread on the bottom of a 13 x 9-inch baking dish. Top with chicken breasts and coat with parmesan cheese.

Bake for 35 to 40 minutes or until chicken is cooked through and no pink remains. Serve over vegetables.

Nutritional Information:

Total calories: 387

Vitamins: Vitamin B6 1.2 μg, Vitamin C 20mg, Phosphorus 475mg, Selenium 46 μg, Niacin 24mg

Sugars: 7g

3.   Superfood Salad

The combination of crisp greens and flaky salmon create the perfect blend of Omega 3 and B vitamins to encourage the best heart function possible. Avocado, blueberry, and pomegranate pack this salad with several essential vitamins!

Ingredients:

- 1/4 cup honey

- 1 tablespoon whole grain mustard

- 1 tablespoons Dijon mustard

- 1 tablespoons extra virgin olive oil

- 1 clove garlic, minced

- 2 (4oz) skinless salmon portions

- 1/2 cup Romaine lettuce, roughly chopped

- 1/2 cup kale, roughly chopped

- 1/2 cup spinach

- 1/2 cup baby arugula

- 1/2 cup fresh blueberries

- 1/2 large avocado, pitted and sliced into strips

- 2 tablespoons pomegranate seeds

- 2 strips nitrate free turkey bacon, cooked and minced

How to prepare:

Whisk together honey, whole grain mustard and Dijon mustard, and garlic together. Pour half into a shallow dish with the salmon portions. Marinate for two hours. Refrigerate remaining half to use as salad dressing.

Lightly spray a skillet with nonstick spray and heat over medium heat. Sauté salmon until cooked through.

In large bowl, toss together romaine, kale, spinach, and arugula with desired amount of dressing. Separate in the servings bowls. Top with blueberries, avocado, pomegranate, bacon, and cooked salmon. Drizzle with additional dressing if desired

Nutritional Information:

Total calories: 416

Vitamins: Vitamin A 138µg, Vitamin B6 0.6mg, Vitamin B12 2.6µg, Vitamin D 8µg, Vitamin K 87µg, Folate 107µg

Minerals: Potassium 980mg, Magnesium 76mg,

Phosphorus 380mg, Selenium 56µg, Niacin 10mg

Sugars 3g

4.   Warm Citrus and Kale Salad

Pairing kale with lemon creates a powerful food combination. Not only does the lemon balance the bold flavor of kale, it combines iron with Vitamin C. This improves absorption of both iron and Vitamin C allowing the body to obtain full benefits of both supplements.

Ingredients:

- 1 tablespoon olive oil
- 1/2 cup zucchini, diced
- 1/2 cup eggplant, diced
- 1/2 cup tomato, diced
- 3 cup kale, chopped
- 1 cup spinach, chopped
- 1/2 cup walnuts, chopped
- 1 tablespoon honey
- 2 tablespoons lemon juice

How to prepare:

In skillet, heat olive oil at medium heat. Add zucchini,

eggplant, and tomato. Cook until soft.

Toss kale and spinach together and divide between serving bowls. Top with zucchini mix and walnuts

In small bowl, whisk together honey and lemon juice. Drizzle over salad and serve.

Nutritional Information:

Total calories: 521

Vitamins: Vitamin A 340µg, Vitamin B6 1mg, Vitamin C 78mg, Vitamin K 431µg

Sugars 7g

5. Summer Spinach Wrap

Celery added to this wrap, or any dish, is a low calorie option with great heart benefit. While not changing the flavor of any recipe, celery boosts oxygen flow in the body, promoting healthy cells and overall heart function.

Ingredients:

- 1 boneless skinless chicken breast, shredded
- 1 medium apple, cubed
- 2 celery stalk, minced
- 2 tablespoons onion, minced
- 3 tablespoons plain Greek yogurt
- 2 teaspoons honey
- 1/2 cup spinach
- 2 large whole wheat tortillas

How to prepare:

Combine all ingredients except spinach and tortilla.

Lay tortillas on flat surface. Divide spinach between both tortillas, top with chicken mixture. Fold in side of tortilla and roll to form burrito shape. Serve.

Nutritional Information:

Total calories: 256

Vitamins: Vitamin B6 0.6mg, Vitamin K 44μg

Minerals: Phosphorus 260mg, Selenium 28μg, Niacin 6mg

Sugars: 15g

6. Blackened Salmon and Bok Choy

Not only is this salmon exploding with spice, it is exploding with Omega 3s and phosphorus. Phosphorus allows healthy heart cells to thrive and remain strong while improving cardiovascular function.

Ingredients:

- 1 tablespoon dried thyme

- 1 teaspoon garlic powder

- 1 teaspoon onion powder

- 1 tablespoon dried oregano

- 1 tablespoon smoked paprika

- 1 teaspoon red pepper

- Kosher or sea salt to taste

- 1 (6 ounce) salmon fillets

- 2 tablespoon olive oil

- 2 green onions, chopped

- 1 tablespoon ginger root, grated

- 2 cloves garlic, grated

- 2 cups bok choy, chopped

- 1 tablespoon water
- 1/2 lime, juiced

How to prepare:

Combine spices in a small bowl. Coat each side of salmon with spice mix. Allow to rest for 5 to 10 minutes. Meanwhile, heat 1 tablespoon olive oil in large skillet on medium heat. Once hot, place salmon skin side up. Cook until fish begins to brown and turns crisp. Carefully turn salmon over and continue to cook second side until crisp. Remove from pan and rest.

In separate medium skillet, heat remaining oil. Add green onion, ginger and garlic. Cook, stirring frequently, until mix begins to brown. Add bok choy and water, continue to cook until bok choy is wilted and water is evaporated. Serve salmon on top of bok choy and drizzled with lime juice.

Nutritional Information:

Total calories: 559

Vitamins: Vitamin B6 0.8mg, Vitamin B12µg, Vitamin D 27µg, Vitamin K 57µg

Sugars: 4g

7. One Skillet Chicken & Pasta

Filled with Vitamin K, this pasta-free lasagna is a brain booster. Vitamin K regulates the calcium in the body improving overall heart health.

Ingredients

- 1/2 pound boneless, skinless chicken breast, chopped into bite-size(1-inch) pieces
- 3 tablespoons extra-virgin olive oil
- 3 cloves garlic, minced
- 1 cup mushrooms, chopped
- 1 cup grape tomatoes, sliced in half
- 10 ounces whole wheat spaghetti, cooked
- 1/4 cup chopped fresh basil leaves
- 3/4 cup grated Parmesan cheese

How to Prepare:

Pour one tablespoon of olive oil in a pot or large skillet over medium heat. Add chicken pieces and mushrooms and cook until chicken is golden and mushrooms softened. Add garlic and tomatoes and cook for one additional minute.

Add remaining ingredients with exception of parmesan. Toss and heat through. Spoon onto serving dishes. Top with parmesan and serve.

Nutritional Information:

Total calories: 381

Vitamins: Vitamin A 272 µg, Vitamin C 98g, Vitamin K 49 µg, Phosphorus 384mg, Niacin 10mg

Sugars: 7g

8. Greek Chicken Salad with Tzatziki Cucumber Dressing

Combine with spinach, walnuts make this a superfood packed salad with Mediterranean flare. Antioxidants protect against degeneration while B vitamins give heart cells energy, promoting healthy blood flow.

Ingredients:

- 4 clove garlic, minced, divided
- 2 teaspoons dry oregano
- 2 tablespoons lemon juice, divided
- 1 tablespoon olive oil
- 2 skinless boneless chicken breast
- 1/2 cup shredded cucumber
- 1 cup Greek yogurt
- 2 teaspoons dry dill
- 4 cups spinach
- 1/4 cup walnuts
- 1/4 cup feta cheese

How to prepare:

Combine 2 cloves of the garlic, oregano, 1 tablespoon lemon juice and olive oil. Pour over chicken breast. Set aside and marinate for 30 minutes. After marinating, cook in skillet on medium heat until internal temperature reaches 165 and no pink remains. Set aside to rest.

In small bowl, combine cucumber (squeezed of excess water), yogurt, dill, remaining garlic, and remaining lemon juice. Mix well.

In two bowls, divide spinach equally. Add 1 tablespoon yogurt dressing into each bowl and toss just until leaves are coated. Top with walnuts, feta cheese and chicken – serve.

Nutritional Information:

Total calories: 452

Vitamins: Vitamin A 319µg, Vitamin B6 1.2mg, Vitamin K 317µg

Minerals: Phosphorus 481mg, Selenium 36µg, Riboflavin 0.5mg, Niacin 10mg

Sugars: 7g

9.   Lentil and Vegetable Soup

Lentils are rich in many vitamins and minerals, too many to list! This key ingredient plays a role in every aspect of heart health – from the aorta to veins and arteries.

Ingredients

- 4 cup low-sodium chicken or vegetable broth
- 1 cup brown lentils, rinsed and raw
- 2 carrots, peeled and chopped
- 2 stalks celery, diced
- 1/2 cup red onion, diced
- 1 bay leaf
- 2 garlic cloves, minced
- 1/2 teaspoon cumin

How to Prepare

Add carrots, celery, and onions to olive oil in the bottom of a medium soup pot on medium heat. Cook until onions are softened and translucent. Add garlic and cook until fragrant. Add broth, lentils, bay leaf, cumin, salt, and pepper.

Bring to a simmer and allow to cook for 25 to 30 minutes, until lentils are cooked through and vegetables have softened. Serve.

Nutritional Information:

Total calories: 575

Vitamins: Vitamin A 346 μg, Vitamin B6, 1.1mg, Vitamin K 152 μg, Phosphorus 660mg, Niacin 11mg

Sugars: 8g

10.   Mushroom and Steak Fajita Pita

High in vitamin E, this mushrooms are the ultimate heart protector. The most potent of all amino acids, vitamin E allows the body to return to normalcy and protects the body and heart from stress while providing energy.

Ingredients

- 1 tablespoon olive oil
- 1 medium red onion, sliced in to strips
- 2 cloves garlic, minced
- 1 medium red bell pepper, cut into strips
- 1-pound beef sirloin tip steak, cut into thin strips
- 1/4 cup mushrooms, sliced
- 2 teaspoons dried oregano
- 1 tablespoon chili powder
- 1/2 teaspoon ground cumin
- 1/4 teaspoon red pepper flakes
- 2 whole wheat pita pockets cut in half
- 4 leaves of Romaine lettuce, torn into small pieces
- 1/4 cup plain Greek yogurt

How to Prepare:

Preheat oven to 350 degrees.

In a large skillet, on medium-low heat, sauté mushrooms in olive oil until soft. Add onions, garlic and bell peppers and continue sautéing until onions and peppers are tender. Add sirloin strips, and cook on medium heat until no longer pink. Sprinkle oregano, chili powder, cumin, and red pepper. Stir well, cover and simmer for 5 minutes. Remove from heat

Stuff pita pockets with meat mixture, romaine lettuce and top with a dollop of yogurt.

Nutritional Information:

Total calories: 580

Vitamins: Vitamin A 389 µg, Vitamin B6 1.4mg, Vitamin B12 2.7 µg, Vitamin K 112 µg, Selenium 70 µg, Zinc 9mg, Niacin 16mg

Sugars: 9g

11.   Avocado Egg Salad

Avocados contain the right combination of healthy fats and vitamins to encourage and improve heart function. Supporting healthy blood flow, avocados also help improve cholesterol and can prevent strokes.

Ingredients

- 1/2 ripe avocado, pitted and peeled
- 1 boiled egg, peeled and chopped
- 2 tablespoons plain Greek yogurt
- 1/4 teaspoon crushed red pepper
- 1 teaspoon fresh parsley, chopped
- 1/4 cup fresh spinach
- 2 slices multigrain bread (toasted, if desired)

How to Prepare

With a fork, smash together all ingredients just until combined Serve between two slices of multigrain bread, top with spinach. Serve.

Nutritional Information:

Total calories: 372

Vitamins: Vitamin B6 0.5mg, Vitamin E 5mg, Vitamin K 176 µg, Selenium 23 µg, Riboflavin 0.5mg

Sugars: 3g

12.   Chicken Salad with Bok Choy, Grapes, and Walnuts

Adding bok choy as a side add extra vitamins in addition to the protein the chicken already contains! Chicken provides more than the minimum amount of daily protein, which is essential to proper heart function.

Ingredients

- 4 ounces boneless skinless chicken breast, cooked and shredded
- 1/4 teaspoon paprika
- 1/4 cup bok choy, diced
- 1 stalk celery, diced
- 1/2 cup diced walnuts
- 12 seedless red grapes, cut in half
- 1/2 cup plain Greek yogurt
- 2 teaspoons honey
- 1/4 teaspoon crushed red pepper
- 4 slices whole grain bread

How to Prepare:

Preheat oven to 325 degrees.

Add walnuts to a small pan, toast in the oven for 10 minutes. Allow to cool.

In a medium bowl combine all ingredients. Mix well.

Lightly toast bread, add chicken salad to two pieces of toast, top with the other two pieces of toast. Cut the two sandwiches in half and serve.

Nutritional Information:

Total calories: 367

Vitamins: Vitamin B6 0,6mg, Selenium 27 µg, Niacin 9mg

Sugars: 16g

13.   Slow Cooker Bean and Potato Soup

Black beans aren't the only bean high in protein, vitamins, and minerals! Cannellini beans and a buttery alternative and provide the same health benefits.

Ingredients

- 3 cups Yukon gold potatoes, peeled and cubed

- 2 cups cannellini beans

- 1/2 cup red onion, chopped

- 2 garlic cloves, minced

- 1/2 cup carrots, chopped

- 1/2 cup celery, chopped

- 2 tablespoons fresh rosemary, minced

- 1/2 tablespoon fresh oregano, minced

- 2 tablespoons fresh thyme, minced

- 1 teaspoon crushed red pepper flakes

- 4 cups chicken bone broth

- 4 tablespoons shredded parmesan cheese

How to Prepare

Add all ingredients to the crockpot, with exception of parmesan, and stir. Allow to cook on low for 8 hours or high for 4 hours. Ladle into serving bowls and sprinkle with parmesan. Serve.

Nutritional Information:

Total calories: 321

Vitamins: Vitamin A 198 µg, Vitamin E 4mg, Phosphorus 252mg, Thiamin 0.6mg

Sugars: 4g

14.   Sweet Potato and Black Bean Burrito

Beta-carotene rich sweet potatoes combined with the perfect protein of black beans and brown rice make this burrito a powerhouse of heart nutrients. The sweet potato has been used to maintain heart health in some of the oldest cultures in the world.

Ingredients:

- 1 sweet potato, peeled and cubed
- 1 tablespoon olive oil
- 1 tablespoon chili powder
- 1 teaspoon ground cumin
- Pinch of Kosher salt
- 4 large whole wheat flour tortillas
- 1/4 cup corn kernels
- 1/2 cup cooked black beans
- 1 cup cooked long grain brown rice
- 1 cup shredded romaine
- 1 yellow pepper, sliced
- 1/2 red onion, sliced
- 1/4 cup salsa

How to prepare:

Preheat oven to 400 degrees.

Toss sweet potato in olive oil, chili powder, cumin, and salt. Place on cooking sheet and roast until potatoes are soft and beginning to brown. About 15 to 20 minutes.

Place tortillas on flat surface, divide potatoes and all other ingredients equally between each tortilla. Fold in side and roll to form burrito. Serve.

Nutritional Information:

Total calories: 317

Vitamins: Vitamin A 337µg, Vitamin B6 0.3mg, Vitamin C 37mg

Minerals: Phosphorus 207mg, Magnesium 6

Mg, Thiamin 0.4mg

Sugars: 6g

15.   Ahi Tuna Tarragon Burger

A great alternative to salmon, Ahi tuna is packed with B Vitamins. The nutrients found in this fish allow for optimal oxygen circulation, providing the heart with all the resources it needs for ultimate heart function.

Ingredients:

- 1/2-pound ahi tuna, minced
- 2 tablespoons onion, minced
- 1 egg
- 3 cloves garlic, minced and divided
- 2 tablespoons ground pistachios
- 1/4 teaspoon cayenne pepper
- 2 tablespoons lime juice, divided
- 1 tablespoon sesame oil
- 1/2 cup plain Greek yogurt
- 2 tablespoons fresh tarragon, chopped
- 1/4 cup shredded cucumber
- 1/2 cup baby arugula
- 2 whole wheat hamburger buns

How to prepare:

Combine tuna, onion, egg, one clove garlic, cayenne pepper, pistachios, and 1 tablespoon lime juice. Form into patties. Patties will be very fragile.

Heat sesame oil in skillet on medium heat. Once hot, place tuna patties in pan and cook until medium and some pink remains (fish can be cooked well-done if desired).

While cooking, combine remaining lime juice, remaining garlic, Greek yogurt, tarragon. Squeeze excess water from cucumber and add to yogurt mixture.

Spread yogurt sauce on to bun, followed by tuna burger. Top with arugula and top bun. Serve.

Nutritional Information:

Total calories: 416

Vitamins: Vitamin B6 1.4mg, Vitamin B12 2.8µg

Minerals: Phosphorus 559mg, Niacin 23mg

Sugars: 7g

16.   Roasted Chicken with Root Vegetables

A blast from the past, this slow cooker chicken is sure to remind anyone of a home cooked Sunday meal. This slow cooking meal is great for a busy lifestyle, ensuring the proper amount of vitamins and minerals.

Ingredients:

- 1 whole chicken
- 1 tablespoon olive oil
- 1 tablespoon fresh sage, minced
- 1 tablespoon fresh rosemary, minced
- 2 clove garlic, minced
- 1 tablespoon fresh thyme, minced
- 1 sweet potato, peeled and cubed
- 1 carrot, peeled and cubed
- 1 turnip, peeled and cubed
- 4 red potatoes, quartered
- 1 small red onion, peeled and cubed
- 2 cups chicken bone broth

How to prepare:

Rub chicken with olive oil, sage, rosemary, thyme and garlic. Place it in slow cooker. Arrange vegetables around chicken and pour broth over vegetables. Cook on low for 8 hours or high for 4 hours until vegetables are tender and no pink remains in chicken. Serve.

Nutritional Information:

Total calories: 333

Vitamins: Vitamin A 371 µg, Vitamin B6 1.3mg, Vitamin B12 0.2 µg, Vitamin C 28mg

Minerals: Phosphorus 359mg, Selenium 30 µg, Zinc 2mg, Niacin 11mg

Sugars: 6g

17.   Nutty Chicken and Roasted Broccolini

A great alternative to everyday fried chicken! Macadamia nuts provide texture, flavor, and protein! In addition to heart health, this nut also benefits the body in many ways, making it a well-rounded nut.

Ingredients:

- 1 cup macadamia nuts, crushed fine
- 2 tablespoons grated parmesan cheese
- 2 tablespoon olive oil, divided
- 2 clove garlic, minced
- 2 small skinless boneless chicken breast
- 3 cups Broccolini florets
- 1 tablespoon fresh basil, chopped

How to prepare:

Heat oven to 400 degrees.

Combine macadamia nuts, parmesan, half the olive oil, and garlic. Place chicken breast on cooking sheet sprayed with nonstick spray, leaving room for Broccolini and press nut topping on to the top and sides of the chicken. Bake for 10 minutes.

Remove pan, and evenly spread Broccolini on reserved pan space with chicken. Drizzle remaining olive oil on Broccolini. Return pan to oven and bake an additional 10 minutes, until no pink remains in chicken and Broccolini is crisp. Plate and serve, sprinkle with fresh basil.

Nutritional Information:

Total calories: 646

Vitamins: Vitamin B6 0.9mg, Vitamin C 79mg, Vitamin K 90 µg

Minerals: Phosphorus 379mg, Selenium 33 µg, Thiamin 0.6mg, Niacin 13mg

Sugars: 4g

18.   Balsamic Chicken with Spinach Apple Salad

Combine with spinach and apple to make this a superfood packed salad with flavor. Antioxidants protect against degeneration while B vitamins give heart cells energy and new life.

Ingredients:

- 2 tablespoon olive oil
- 2 (6 ounce) boneless, skinless chicken breasts
- 2 tablespoons balsamic vinegar
- 2 green onions, diced
- 1 green apple, sliced into thin wedges
- 1 stalk celery, diced
- 1 tablespoon lemon juice
- 2 cups baby spinach
- 1 tablespoon honey

How to Prepare:

Heat olive oil in a large skillet over medium heat. Cook until golden brown and cooked through, with no pink remaining.

Remove from heat and add the vinegar. Turn the chicken to coat.

In a large bowl, toss the green onion, apple, celery, and lemon juice. Fold in the spinach top with the chicken and drizzle with honey.

Nutritional Information:

Total calories: 373

Vitamins: Vitamin B6 1.2mg, Vitamin K 209 µg, Phosphorus 437mg, Selenium 46 µg, Niacin 23mg

Sugars: 17g

19. Roasted Salmon and Sundried Tomato Green Beans

This may be the simplest of recipes, packed with flavor and an abundance of vitamins and minerals. With over daily recommendations of Vitamin B12, Vitamin D, and Niacin, this easy recipe will boost your heart's abilities!

Ingredients:

- 6 clove garlic, minced
- 1 pound green beans, trimmed
- 1/4 cup sundried tomatoes, chopped
- 2 tablespoons olive oil
- 2 (8 ounces) salmon fillet

How to Prepare:

Heat oven to 425 degrees F. On a large rimmed baking sheet, toss together the garlic, beans, tomatoes, and 1 tablespoon olive oil. Roast for about 15 minute, or until tender and beginning to brown.

Meanwhile, heat the remaining tablespoon oil in a large skillet over medium heat. Cook salmon until golden brown and opaque throughout, 4 to 5 minutes per side. Serve with the vegetables.

Nutritional Information:

Total calories: 602

Vitamins: Vitamin A 288 µg, Vitamin B6 2.5mg, Vitamin B12 19.1 µg, Vitamin D 44 µg Magnesium 196mg Riboflavin 0.7mg

Sugars: 12g

20. Seared Tuna with Cucumber Pineapple Relish

Take a break from salmon and kick Vitamin B into high gear with Ahi Tuna! A great alternative to salmon, Ahi tuna contains enough Vitamin B to give you extra energy and improve heart function.

Ingredients:

- 2 cups brown rice, cooked
- 2 tablespoons lime juice
- 1 tablespoon fresh ginger, grated
- 2 teaspoons honey
- 2 tablespoons olive oil
- 2 green onions, chopped
- 1 jalapeño pepper, minced
- 1 cup fresh pineapple, chopped
- 1/2 cup cucumber, chopped
- 2 (8 ounces) tuna filets

How to Prepare:

In a large bowl, whisk together the lime juice, ginger,

honey, and half the oil. Toss with the scallions, jalapeño, pineapple and cucumber.

Heat the remaining oil in a large nonstick skillet over medium heat. Add tuna and cook until firm, but still pink in the middle. Serve cucumber pineapple relish over tuna and rice.

Nutritional Information:

Total calories: 472

Vitamins: Vitamin B6 1.8mg, Vitamin B12 3.3 µg, Vitamin C 86mg, Magnesium 126mg, Niacin 32mg

Sugars: 11g

21.   Rice and Black Bean Salad

A great low carb entrée! The blend of black beans and brown rice not only combine to make a perfect protein, but make this little salad a filling meal.

Ingredients

- 3 tablespoons lime juice
- 2 tablespoons olive oil
- ½ teaspoon. ground cumin
- 2 cups brown rice, cooked
- 1 cup black beans, cooked
- 2 cups romaine lettuce, chopped
- 1 tablespoon fresh cilantro, chopped
- 1/2 cup corn
- 1/2 cup tomato, diced
- 1 cup avocado, diced
- 1/4 cup red onion, diced
- 2 tablespoons plain Greek yogurt

How to Prepare:

In a small bowl, whisk together the lime juice, oil and cumin.

Divide the rice and beans among serving bowls. Top with the lettuce, cilantro, corn, tomatoes, avocado, and onion.

Drizzle with lime juice mix and top with Greek yogurt. Serve.

Nutritional Information:

Total calories: 315

Vitamins: Vitamin A 113 μg, Vitamin C 28mg, Vitamin K 45 μg, Phosphorus 232mg

Sugars: 2g

22.　Chickpea and Red Pepper Soup

A great fall soup, red peppers are perfect for a cool day. Chickpeas make this a well-rounded dish and gives this soup a boost of protein.

Ingredients:

- 1/2 cup quinoa, cooked
- 2 tablespoons olive oil
- 1 medium onion, chopped
- 1 carrot, chopped
- 2 stalk celery, chopped
- 3 clove garlic, minced
- 1 tablespoon smoked paprika
- 2 red pepper, chopped
- 2 cups chickpeas, cooked
- 2 cups vegetable broth
- 1 cup water
- 2 tablespoons red wine vinegar

How to Prepare:

Heat the oil in a large pot. Add the onion, carrot, and celery and cook, covered, stirring occasionally, until onion is softened

Add the garlic and paprika, stirring until fragment. Add the red peppers and cook, stirring occasionally, for 5 minutes.

Add the chickpeas, broth, and water and bring to a boil. Reduce heat and simmer until the vegetables are tender. Stir in the vinegar and cooked quinoa. Ladle into bowls and serve.

Nutritional Information:

Total calories: 605

Vitamins: Vitamin A 767 µg, Vitamin K 52 µg, Phosphorus 618mg, Riboflavin 0.6mg

Sugars: 21g

23.   Avocado Crab Salad

The healthy fats in the avocado combined with B Vitamins and Omega 3s make the salad a balanced heart healthy meal. Can be served as an appetizer or main entrée.

Ingredients:

- 2 avocados, diced small
- 1 teaspoon lemon zest
- 1 tablespoon lemon juice
- 2 cups lump crab meat
- 2 tablespoon radish, minced
- 3 tablespoon plain Greek yogurt
- 1 tablespoon fresh basil, chopped

How to Prepare:

Combine all ingredients and mix well. Serve with grilled or toasted pita bread or as a sandwich.

Nutritional Information:

Total calories: 569

Vitamins: Vitamin B6 0.5mg, Vitamin B12 3.6 µg, Vitamin K 108 µg Selenium 47 µg

Sugars: 2g

24.   Horseradish Salmon Cakes

A zesty favorite, horseradish also provides a punch of Vitamin C and cuts the fatty texture of the salmon – which is packed with Vitamin B and Omega-3s.

Ingredients:

- 2 (8 ounce) salmon fillet
- 2 tablespoons horseradish, minced well
- 1 tablespoon Dijon mustard
- 1/4 cup whole wheat panko bread crumbs
- 2 tablespoons olive oil
- 2 tablespoons plain Greek yogurt
- 1 tablespoon lemon juice

How to prepare:

In a food processor, pulse the salmon, horseradish, mustard, until coarsely chopped. Mix in panko and form the mixture into 8 patties.

Heat half the oil in a large nonstick skillet over medium heat. Cook the patties until firm until no pink remains.

In a large bowl, whisk together the yogurt, lemon juice, remaining and oil. Top patties with yogurt mix and serve.

Nutritional Information:

Total calories: 792

Vitamins: Vitamin B6, 1.1mg, Vitamin B12 6.7 µg, Vitamin D 19 µg Phosphorus 824mg

Sugars: 3g

25.   Bacon Spinach and Sweet Potato Quiche

Quick and easy heart food to start a busy day. Sweet potato makes this quiche flavorful and filling. Packed with Vitamin A and C it's the perfect balance of delicious and nutritious.

Ingredients

- 2 cups sweet potato, grated
- 1 teaspoon olive oil
- 1 yellow onion, diced
- 6 slices turkey bacon, thinly sliced
- 1 cup spinach chopped
- 1/2 teaspoon dried dill
- 2 large eggs
- 4 large egg whites
- 1/4 cup skim milk
- 1/4 cup feta cheese

How to Prepare:

Preheat oven to 400 degrees.

Coat a 9-inch pie plate with cooking spray. Gently press the sweet potato into the bottom of the pie plate and up the sides, forming a pie crust. Place in the oven and bake until sweet potato crust is cooked, about 20 minutes. Remove from oven and decrease oven temperate to 350 degrees.

In a medium pan, warm oil over medium-high heat. Add onion and cook until translucent. Add turkey bacon, continuing to stir and cook until onions and bacon begin to brown. Stir in spinach, and dill; cook until water from the spinach is wilted and transfer mixture from pan into the sweet potato pie shell.

In a bowl, add eggs, egg whites, and milk. Using a fork, whisk to combine. Pour eggs over vegetable mixture in the pie shell. Sprinkle the feta cheese over the top of quiche.

Cook quiche in oven until eggs in the center are set, about 35 to 40 minutes. Remove from oven and let cool just a few minutes before slicing. Serve.

Nutritional Information:

Total calories: 422

Vitamins: Vitamin A 443 µg, Vitamin K 164 µg, Selenium 16 µg, Phosphorus 283mg

Sugars: 3g

26.   Curry Stuffed Bell Peppers

A great low carb alternative to a traditional stuffed pepper! The blend of curry and vegetables not only combine to make a well-rounded entree, but make this little pepper a filling meal.

Ingredients

- 4 medium bell peppers, tops cut off, seeds and white membrane removed
- 1 tablespoon olive oil
- 1 small onion, diced
- 1-pound ground turkey
- 1 cup zucchini, diced
- 1 teaspoon curry powder
- 1 teaspoon honey
- 1/2 teaspoon ground cloves
- 1/2 teaspoon garlic powder
- 1 cup chicken bone broth
- 1 1/2 cups quinoa, cooked
- 2 tablespoons fresh cilantro, chopped

How to Prepare:

Preheat oven to 375 degrees

In a large skillet, heat oil over medium heat. Add onions and cook until translucent. Add ground chicken - breaking up clumps and stirring until cooked through. Add zucchini, curry powder, honey, cloves, and garlic powder. Stir and cook until fragrant.

Stir in chicken broth, quinoa, and cilantro until well mixed. Spoon mixture in to each bell pepper. Place peppers in an 8x8 baking dish, standing up. Add enough water to cover the bottom of the baking.

Bake 25-30 minutes in preheated oven until peppers are tender and mixture is heated through. Serve.

27. Herb Flank Steak

Not only do fresh herbs add flavor to any dish, but they're packed with nutrients! Vitamins E and K, found in fresh herbs, paired with steak make this a filling and nutritious entrée.

Ingredients

- 1 teaspoon fresh thyme, chopped

- 1 teaspoon fresh oregano, chopped

- 1 teaspoon fresh parsley, chopped

- 2 teaspoons olive oil

- 1/4 teaspoon lemon zest

- 1 garlic clove, minced

- 1-pound flank steak

- 1/4 cup red wine vinegar

- 1/4 cup beef bone broth

How to Prepare:

Preheat oven to 400 degrees.

Combine thyme, oregano, oil, lemon zest, and garlic in a

small bowl; set aside.

Heat a large ovenproof skillet over medium-high heat. Add steak to pan; cook 1 minute on each side or until browned. Add wine and broth; cook 1 minute. Spread herb mixture over steak; place pan in oven. Bake for 10 minutes or until desired degree of doneness. Let stand 10 minutes before cutting steak diagonally across the grain into thin slices.

Nutritional Information:

Total calories: 456

Vitamins: Vitamin C 93mg, Magnesium 20mg, Niacin 10mg

Sugars: 3g

28.   Peanut Chicken Stir Fry

A light meal option, this chicken salad sandwich contains selenium. Acting as an antioxidant, selenium repairs nerve cells preventing cardiovascular decline.

Ingredients

- 1 cup long-grain brown rice, cooked
- 2 cups chicken breast, cooked and shredded
- 1/2 cup shredded carrot
- 1/3 cup green onions, sliced
- 1/4 cup dry-roasted peanuts, divided
- 1 tablespoon fresh cilantro, chopped
- 2 tablespoons fresh lime juice
- 4 teaspoons olive oil
- 1 teaspoon sesame oil
- 2 garlic cloves, minced

How to Prepare:

Combine rice, chicken, carrot, onions, 2 tablespoons peanuts, teaspoons cilantro and lime juice; toss to combine.

In skillet on medium heat, heat oil. Add rice mix and cook stirring frequently until rice begins to brown and ingredients are heated through. Serve.

Nutritional Information:

Total calories: 456

Vitamins: Vitamin C 112mg, Magnesium 111mg, Niacin 10mg

Sugars: 3g

29. Cilantro Lime Chicken

Spices such as cilantro are loaded with Vitamin C, making this citrus inspired entrée extra beneficial. The highest levels of Vitamin C are found in tissues around the heart. Allow this chicken dish to boost heart function.

Ingredients

- 2 tablespoons fresh cilantro, chopped
- 2 tablespoons fresh lime juice
- 1 tablespoons olive oil
- 4 (6-ounce) skinless, boneless chicken breast
- 1 cup tomato, chopped
- 2 tablespoons onion, minced
- 2 teaspoons lime juice
- 1 avocado, peeled and finely chopped

How to Prepare:

In a large bowl combine cilantro, lime and chicken. Cover and refrigerate for one hour.

Heat skillet over medium heat. Add chicken and cook

through until no pink remains.

In small bowl, combine remaining ingredients. Toss to combine. Serve on top of chicken.

Nutritional Information:

Total calories: 472

Vitamins: Vitamin B6 1.8mg, Vitamin B12 3.3 µg, Vitamin C 86mg, Magnesium 126mg, Niacin 32mg

Sugars: 11g

30.   Peanut Crusted Chicken

Change up every day chicken with the creamy flavor of peanut. Peanuts give this classic dish added depth and flavor. The antioxidants in peanuts help maintain collagen in arteries and veins, keeping them functioning properly.

Ingredients

- 1 cup fresh pineapple, chopped
- 1 tablespoon fresh cilantro, chopped
- 1 tablespoon red onion, minced
- 1/3 cup unsalted, dry-roasted peanuts
- 1 cup panko bread crumbs
- 4 (4-ounce) boneless skinless chicken breast
- 1 tablespoon olive oil

How to Prepare:

In small bowl, combine pineapple, cilantro, and red onion. Toss well and set aside.

Combine peanuts and panko in a food processor; process until finely chopped. Dredge chicken in the breadcrumb mixture.

Heat oil in a large nonstick skillet over medium-high heat. Add chicken to pan, cook through until no pink remains. Serve chicken with pineapple mixture.

Nutritional Information:

Total calories: 792

Vitamins: Vitamin B6, 1.1mg, Vitamin B12 6.7 µg, Vitamin D 19 µg Phosphorus 824mg

Sugars: 6g

31.　Cashew Chicken Stir Fry

Chicken goes with everything, and adding cashews is an amazing combination! The crunch and earthiness provides and out of this world experience sure to fulfill every vitamin and mineral needed.

Ingredients

- 2 tablespoons hoisin sauce, divided
- 1 teaspoon rice wine vinegar
- 3/4 teaspoon honey
- 1/2 teaspoon crushed red pepper
- 1-pound chicken breast tenders, cut into thin strips
- 1/2 cup coarsely chopped unsalted cashews
- 2 tablespoons olive oil
- 2 cups red pepper, sliced
- 1 clove garlic, minced
- 1 teaspoon fresh ginger, grated
- 2 green onions, chopped

How to Prepare:

Heat oil in medium skillet. Add garlic and ginger and cook until fragrant. Add chicken, cook through until no pink remains. Add remaining ingredients and cook until peppers and onions are slightly soft. Serve over brown rice or quinoa.

Nutritional Information:

Total calories: 317

Vitamins: Vitamin A 337µg, Vitamin B6 0.3mg, Vitamin C 37mg

Minerals: Phosphorus 207mg, Magnesium 6Mg, Thiamin 0.4mg

Sugars: 6g

32.   Mediterranean Turkey Burger

A spin on the popular Mediterranean diet, this burger is overflowing with flavor. Popular Mediterranean spices, such as garlic and feta, provide extra nutrients to improve cardiovascular function.

Ingredients

- 1/4 cup crumbled feta cheese

- 1 tablespoon red onion, minced

- 2 tablespoons basil pesto

- 1-pound ground turkey breast

- 1 garlic clove, minced

- 2 cups arugula

- 2 whole-wheat pitas, toasted and halved

How to Prepare:

Combine all ingredients with the exception of arugula and pita. Form mix into patties. Grill or sear until cook through and no pink remains.

Place burgers between two slices of pita and top with

arugula. Serve.

Nutritional Information:

Total calories: 472

Vitamins: Vitamin B6 1.8mg, Vitamin B12 3.3 µg, Vitamin C 86mg, Magnesium 126mg, Niacin 32mg

Sugars: 11g

33.   Chicken and White Bean Chili

This well rounded chili is a great source of iron. Iron is directly connected to heart health and functions. Not only does iron assist in proper blood flow, it creates pathways to help with the prevention of cardiovascular decline.

Ingredients

- 1 tablespoon olive oil

- 2 cups onion, diced

- 1 tablespoons chili powder

- 2 clove garlic, minced

- 1 teaspoons ground cumin

- 1 teaspoon dried oregano

- 3 cups cannellini beans

- 4 cups chicken bone broth

- 3 cups skinless boneless chicken breast, chopped

- 1 (14 ounce) can diced tomatoes

How to Prepare:

Combine all ingredients in slow cooker. Cook on high for 4

hours or low for 8 hours.

Remove chicken and shred. Return to slow cooker. Cover and cook and additional 30 minutes. Serve.

Nutritional Information:

Total calories: 456

Vitamins: Vitamin C 93mg, Magnesium 20mg, Niacin 10mg

Sugars: 3g

34.   Seared Salmon with Apple Slaw

This may be the simplest of recipes, packed with flavor and an abundance of vitamins and minerals. With over daily recommendations of Vitamin B12, Vitamin D, and Niacin, this easy recipe will boost your hearts every day abilities!

Ingredients:

- 1 teaspoon olive oil
- 2 (8 ounce) salmon filets
- kosher salt and black pepper
- 2 cups bok choy, thinly sliced
- 1 red apple, shredded
- 4 green onions, thinly sliced
- 1/3 cup plain Greek yogurt
- 1 teaspoon honey
- 2 tablespoons fresh lemon juice

How to Prepare:

Heat the oil in a large nonstick skillet over medium-high heat. Sear the salmon cook until firm and flaky.

Meanwhile, in a medium bowl, toss remaining ingredients. Spoon onto plate and place salmon on top. Serve.

Nutritional Information:

Total calories: 333

Vitamins: Vitamin A 371 µg, Vitamin B6 1.3mg, Vitamin B12 1.2 µg, Vitamin C 28mg

Minerals: Phosphorus 359mg, Selenium 30 µg, Zinc 2mg, Niacin 11mg

Sugars: 6g

35. Southwest Black Bean Stuffed Bell Pepper

A great low carb alternative to a traditional southwest cuisine! The blend of black beans and brown rice combine to make a perfect protein, providing the cardiovascular system the nutrients it needs to function.

Ingredients:

- 2 large red bell peppers
- 1 tablespoon olive oil, divided
- 1 clove garlic, minced
- 1 small onion, chopped
- 1 cup black beans, cooked
- 1 cup cooked brown rice
- 2 cups salsa, preferably homemade
- 1/4 cup fresh cilantro, chopped
- 1/4 cup shredded cheddar cheese

How to prepare:

Preheat oven to 375 degrees.

Cut off the tops of the peppers, carefully scoop out the seeds and white ribs creating a bowl. Place on cookie sheet sprayed with nonstick spray.

Heat olive oil in large sauté pan over medium heat and add onions and garlic. Mix in beans, rice, and salsa. Cook until warmed though.

Spoon mixture into peppers and top with cheese. Bake 20 to 25 minutes, until peppers are soft and filling is hot.

Nutritional Information:

Total calories: 536

Vitamins: Vitamin A 325µg, Vitamin B6 1.1mg, Vitamin C 261mg, Vitamin E 8mg, Vitamin K 44µg

Minerals: Magnesium 138mg, Phosphorus 387mg, Folate 180µg, Thiamin 0.5mg

Sugars: 15g

36.   Asian Halibut

Combining Halibut and ginger in this crisp fresh entrée create a super force of heart boosting vitamins and minerals. Red cabbage is a powerful antiaging source while Halibut is packed with OMEGA3s and B Vitamins to give the heart extra energy.

Ingredients:

- 1 tablespoon lime juice

- 1 teaspoon fresh ginger, grated

- 2 tablespoons olive oil

- 1 cup red pepper, sliced

- 1 small red onion, thinly sliced

- 1 tablespoon sesame seeds, toasted

- 2 (6-ounce) pieces halibut fillet

How to Prepare:

In a large bowl, combine the lime juice, ginger, 1 tablespoon of the oil, red pepper, onion, and sesame seeds, and toss to coat.

Heat the remaining tablespoon of oil in a large nonstick skillet over medium-high heat. Add halibut and cook until translucent, firm and flaky. Transfer to serving plate and top with veggies. Serve.

Nutritional Information:

Total calories: 416

Vitamins: Vitamin B6 1.4mg, Vitamin B12 2.8μg

Minerals: Phosphorus 559mg, Niacin 23mg

Sugars: 7g

37.   Fennel Stuffed Chicken and balsamic tomatoes

Fennel and tomato ensure this chicken dish contains vitamin C while chicken provide selenium helps to maintain heart health.

Ingredients:

- 2 tablespoons fresh thyme leaves
- 4 (6-ounce) boneless, skinless chicken breasts
- 2 tablespoons olive oil
- 2 tomatoes, diced
- 1 shallot, thinly sliced
- 1 tablespoon red wine vinegar
- 1 fennel bulb, sliced

How to Prepare:

Preheat oven to 400 degrees.

Heat oil in skillet on medium heat, add fennel and thyme leaves. Cook until fennel is sliced. Cut a 2-inch pocket in the thickest part of each chicken breast. Stuff cooked fennel into pocket. Place on nonstick cooking sheet and bake, 15

– 20 minutes until cooked though and chicken is no longer pink.

Mix the tomatoes, shallot, and vinegar in small bowl. Slice the chicken, if desired, and serve with the tomato salad.

Nutritional Information:

Total calories: 315

Vitamins: Vitamin A 210 µg, Vitamin B6 0.5mg, Vitamin B12 0.9 µg, Vitamin K 98µg

Minerals: Calcium 444mg, Potassium 1050mg, Riboflavin 0.5mg, Niacin 6mg

Sugars: 15g

38.   Southern Chicken and Collard Greens

Leafy greens are loaded with Vitamin C, making this Southern inspired entrée extra beneficial. The highest levels of Vitamin C are found in the heart tissues where heart energy is most frequently used.

Ingredients:

- 2 tablespoons olive oil

- 4 (6-ounce) boneless, skinless chicken breasts

- 2 teaspoons blackening or Cajun seasoning

- 4 cloves garlic, minced

- 1 red bell pepper, chopped

- 2 cups collard greens, sliced

- 1 cup black-eyed peas, cooked

How to Prepare:

Heat 1 tablespoon of the oil in a large skillet over medium heat. Season the chicken with blackening seasoning, cook the chicken until golden brown and cooked through, with no pink remaining. Transfer to plates.

Meanwhile, in a second skillet, heat the remaining oil over medium-high heat. Add the garlic and bell pepper to the second skillet and cook, tossing frequently, until beginning to soften. Add the collard greens, cook, tossing, until just tender, stir in the black-eyed peas and cook until heated through. Serve with chicken.

Nutritional Information:

Total calories: 589

Vitamins: Vitamin B6 0.5mg, Vitamin E 3mg, Vitamin K 50µg

Minerals: Magnesium 132mg, Phosphorus 433mg, Selenium 85µg, Zinc 4mg

Sugars: 6g

39.   Middle Eastern Lamb with Saffron Rice

Lamb is not just for special occasions! Lamb is an outstanding source of zinc, iron, and Vitamin B12 and should be eaten more often.

Ingredients:

- 1 cup long-grain brown rice

- 1 teaspoon curry powder

- 2 tablespoons fresh basil, chopped

- 1 tablespoon olive oil

- 1 tablespoon lemon juice

- 2 clove garlic, minced

- 8 small rib or loin lamb chops

How to Prepare:

Cook the rice according to the package directions, adding curry powder to the water before cooking. Once cooked, fold in basil.

Meanwhile, heat the oil in a large skillet over medium-high heat. Add garlic and cook until fragrant. Add lamb and cook until firm, slightly pink in middle. Serve the lamb over rice. Drizzle with lemon juice.

Nutritional Information:

Total calories: 617

Vitamins: Vitamin A 337µg, Vitamin B6 0.3mg, Vitamin C 37mg

Minerals: Phosphorus 207mg, Magnesium 6

Mg, Thiamin 0.4mg

Sugars: 6g

40.   Honey Glazed Salmon with Ginger Spinach

Combining honey and spinach is a classic combination. Honey sweetens the earthiness of the spinach; not only creating a balance of flavor and a well-rounded dish rich in vitamins and minerals.

Ingredients:

- 1 tablespoon honey
- 3 teaspoons Hoisin sauce
- 2 (8 ounce) salmon filets
- 1 tablespoon olive oil
- 1 red bell pepper, thinly sliced
- 1 tablespoon chopped fresh ginger
- 3 cups spinach, chopped
- 1 tablespoon toasted sesame seeds

How to Prepare:

Heat broiler. In a small bowl, combine the honey and 1 teaspoon of the Hoisin sauce.

Place the salmon on a foil-lined broiler-proof baking sheet.

Broil for 5 minutes. Spoon the honey mixture over the salmon and broil until the salmon is firm and flaky.

Meanwhile, heat the oil in a large skillet over medium-high heat. Add the bell pepper and cook, tossing occasionally, until just tender, stir in the ginger.

Add the spinach and cook until just wilted. Add the remaining 2 teaspoons of Hoisin sauce. Serve with the salmon and sprinkle with the sesame seeds.

Nutritional Information:

Total calories: 441

Vitamins: Vitamin A 216µg, Vitamin B6 1.2mg, Vitamin C 82mg, Vitamin K 183µg

Minerals: Niacin 14mg, Magnesium 115mg, Phosphorus 397mg, Selenium 32µg

Sugars: 9g

41. Chicken and White Bean Stew

A great fall soup, chicken and white beans soup is earthy and perfect for a cool day. A variety of vegetables make this a well-rounded dish while chicken gives this soup a boost of protein.

Ingredients:

- 1 tablespoon extra-virgin olive oil, divided
- 1/2 cup carrot, diced
- 1 (8 ounce) boneless, skinless chicken breast, cut into quarters
- 1 clove garlic, minced
- 5 cups chicken bone broth
- 1 teaspoon dried marjoram
- 2 cups spinach, chopped
- 1 cup cannellini beans
- 1/4 cup grated Parmesan cheese
- 1/3 cup fresh basil, chopped

How to Prepare:

Heat half oil in large saucepan over medium-high heat. Add carrot and chicken; cook, turning the chicken and stirring frequently, until the chicken begins to brown. Add garlic and cook until fragrant. Stir in broth and marjoram; bring to a boil over high heat. Reduce the heat and simmer, stirring occasionally, until the chicken is cooked through.

With a slotted spoon, transfer the chicken pieces to a clean cutting board to cool. Add spinach and beans to the pot and bring to a gentle boil.

Combine the remaining oil, Parmesan and basil in a food processor. Process until a coarse paste forms, adding a little water and scraping down the sides if necessary.

Cut the chicken into bite-size pieces. Stir the chicken and pesto into the pot. Heat until hot. Spoon into bowls and serve.

Nutritional Information:

Total calories: 441

Vitamins: Vitamin A 216µg, Vitamin B6 1.2mg, Vitamin C 82mg, Vitamin K 183µg

Minerals: Niacin 14mg, Magnesium 115mg, Phosphorus 397mg, Selenium 32µg

Sugars: 9g

42.　Penne Lasagna Bowl

Filled with Vitamin K, this lasagna is a heart booster. Vitamin K regulates the calcium in the blood improving overall cardiovascular health.

Ingredients:

- 8 ounces whole-wheat rotini, cooked
- 1 tablespoon olive oil
- 1 onion, chopped
- 3 cloves garlic, minced
- 1 cup mushrooms, sliced
- 1 14-ounce diced can tomatoes with Italian herbs
- 2 cups spinach, chopped
- 1/2 teaspoon crushed red pepper
- 3/4 cup ricotta cheese

How to Prepare:

Heat oil in a large nonstick skillet over medium heat. Add onion and garlic and cook, stirring, until soft and beginning to brown, add mushrooms, and cook, stirring, until the mushrooms release their liquid.

Add tomatoes, spinach and crushed red pepper. Cook until the spinach is wilted.

Toss the sauce with the pasta and divide among 4 bowls. Dollop each serving with ricotta.

Nutritional Information:

Total calories: 518

Vitamins: Vitamin A 137µg, Vitamin B6 1.3mg, Vitamin C 26mg, Vitamin K 125µg,

Minerals: Niacin 14mg, Phosphorus 420mg, Selenium 46µg, Zinc 3mg

Sugars: 24g

43.   Sundried Tomato Chicken and Orzo

A powerhouse of anti-inflammatory agents, this sundried tomato dish increases blood flow and provides heart cells with the oxygen they need, each of these ingredients should be consumed on a regular basis.

Ingredients:

- 8 ounces orzo, preferably whole-wheat, cooked
- 1 cup water
- 1/2 cup chopped sun-dried tomatoes
- 1 clove garlic, minced
- 3 teaspoons fresh marjoram, chopped
- 1 tablespoon red-wine vinegar
- 1 tablespoon olive oil, divided
- 4 boneless, skinless chicken breasts
- 1/4 cup grated parmesan cheese

How to Prepare:

Place sun-dried tomatoes, water, garlic, marjoram, vinegar and 1/2 oil in a blender. Blend until just a few chunks remain. Add water if needed.

Heat remaining oil in a large skillet over medium-high heat. Add the chicken and cook, until golden outside and no longer pink in the middle. Remove from heat and keep warm.

Pour the blended tomato sauce into the pan and bring to a boil. Add orzo and cook, stirring, until heated through. Divide onto plates and top with cheese.

Slice the chicken. Top each portion of pasta with sliced chicken.

Nutritional Information:

Total calories: 532

Vitamins: Vitamin A 413µg, B-6 0.6mg, B-12 1.4µg, Vitamin C 76mg, Vitamin K 300µg

Minerals: Copper 850 µg, Iron 4mg, Magnesium 97mg, Niacin 9mg, Phosphorus 599mg, Selenium 46µg, Zinc 4mg

Sugars 12g

44.   Almond Crusted Chicken

A great alternative to everyday fried chicken! Almonds provide texture, flavor, and protein! Protein gives you arteries and heart strength.

Ingredients:

- 1/2 cup sliced almonds
- 1/4 cup whole-wheat flour
- 1 1/2 teaspoons paprika
- 1/2 teaspoon garlic powder
- 1/2 teaspoon dry mustard
- 1/4 teaspoon salt
- 1/8 teaspoon freshly ground pepper
- 1 1/2 teaspoons extra-virgin olive oil
- 4 large egg whites
- 1-pound chicken tenders

How to Prepare:

Preheat oven to 475 degrees. Line a baking sheet with foil and spray with nonstick cooking spray.

Place almonds, flour, paprika, garlic powder, dry mustard, salt and pepper in a food processor; process until the almonds are finely chopped and the paprika is mixed throughout. With the motor running, drizzle in oil; process until combined. Transfer the mixture to a shallow dish.

Whisk egg whites in a second shallow dish. Add chicken tenders and turn to coat. Transfer each tender to the almond mixture; turn to coat evenly. Place the tenders on the prepared baking sheet.

Bake the chicken fingers until golden brown, crispy and no longer pink in the center, 20 to 25 minutes.

Nutritional Information:

Total calories: 518

Vitamins: Vitamin A 137µg, Vitamin B6 1.3mg, Vitamin C 26mg, Vitamin K 125µg,

Minerals: Niacin 14mg, Phosphorus 420mg, Selenium 46µg, Zinc 3mg

Sugars: 24g

45. Maple Dijon Chicken

Dijon gives this chicken a kick with maple gives this entrée a balanced sweetness. This chicken is loaded with minerals to keep the heart pumping.

Ingredients:

- 3 tablespoons Dijon mustard
- 2 tablespoons maple syrup
- 2 tablespoons olive oil, divided
- 1 tablespoon fresh thyme, chopped
- 2 (8 ounce) boneless skinless chicken breasts

How to Prepare:

Whisk mustard, maple syrup, 1 tablespoon oil, thyme, pepper and salt in a large bowl. Add chicken and turn to coat evenly. Cover and marinate in the refrigerator for at least 30 minutes and up to 6 hours.

Preheat oven to 400 degrees. Cover baking sheet with foil and spray with nonstick spray. Arrange chicken on sheet.

Bake until golden brown and cooked through. Serve.

Nutritional Information:

Total calories: 229

Vitamins: Vitamin A 178µg, Vitamin B6 0.4mg, Vitamin B12 1.5µg, Vitamin C 26mg, Vitamin K 113µg

Minerals: Phosphorus 365mg, Selenium 54µg, Magnesium 32mg

Sugars 4g

46.   Fettuccini and Brussel Sprouts

A quick week night option, this fettuccini and Brussel sprouts is a wonderful change from day to day dinners. Not typically a favorite, if made correctly Brussels sprouts are better than popcorn, not only in flavor but in numerous Vitamins and Minerals!

Ingredients:

- 12 ounces whole-wheat fettuccine, cooked
- 1 tablespoon olive oil
- 4 cups mushrooms, sliced
- 4 cups thinly sliced Brussels sprouts
- 1 tablespoon minced garlic
- 2 tablespoons sherry vinegar
- 1 cup low-fat milk
- 1 cup grated parmesan cheese

How to Prepare:

Heat oil in a large skillet over medium heat. Add mushrooms and Brussels sprouts and cook, stirring often, until the mushrooms release their liquid. Add garlic and cook, stirring, until fragrant. Add sherry vinegar, scraping up any brown bits; bring to a boil and cook, stirring, until almost evaporated.

Add milk to the skillet bring to a boil. Lower heat and stir in cheese until thickened. Add the sauce to the pasta; gently toss. Serve.

Nutritional Information:

Vitamins: Vitamin B6 .4mg, Vitamin B12 1µg

Minerals: Phosphorus 280mg, Selenium 32µg, Niacin 6mg, Zinc 3mg, Riboflavin 0.3mg

Sugars 3g

47.   Sweet and Spicy Salmon

A perfect balance of creamy and cool. Salmon provides healthy fats and Vitamin B, keeping the heart healthy and functioning to the best of its ability.

Ingredients

- 3 tablespoons honey
- 1 tablespoon Hoisin sauce
- 4 teaspoons hot mustard
- 1 teaspoon rice vinegar
- 4 (6-ounce) salmon fillets

How to Prepare:

Preheat oven to 425 degrees

Combine honey, Hoisin sauce, mustard, and rice vinegar in small sauce pot. Bring to a boil.

Place fish on a foil-lined baking pan coated with nonstick cooking spray. Bake for 12 minutes and remove from oven.

Preheat broiler.

Brush sauce evenly over salmon; broil for 3 minutes or until firm and flaky. Serve.

Nutritional Information:

Total calories: 518

Vitamins: Vitamin A 137µg, Vitamin B6 1.3mg, Vitamin C 26mg, Vitamin K 125µg,

Minerals: Niacin 14mg, Phosphorus 420mg, Selenium 46µg, Zinc 3mg

Sugars: 24g

48.   Herb Crusted Turkey Breast

Not only do fresh herbs add flavor to any dish, but they're packed with nutrients! Vitamins E and K, found in fresh herbs, paired with turkey breast make this a well-rounded chicken alternative.

Ingredients:

- 1pound turkey breast half with skin, thawed if frozen
- 3 tablespoon lime juice
- 2 tablespoon olive oil
- 4 clove garlic, minced
- 1 teaspoon dried oregano
- 1/2 teaspoon dried tarragon
- 1/2 teaspoon crushed red pepper

How to Prepare:

Pre heat oven to 325 degrees. Lightly spray a large glass baking dish with cooking spray. Place turkey in the baking dish.

In a small bowl, stir together the remaining ingredients.

Spread the mixture as evenly as possible over the turkey.

Roast turkey, covered, for 20 minutes. Uncover and continue to roast until cooked through and no pink remains. Allow to rest for 10 minutes. Slice and serve.

Nutritional Information:

Total calories: 518

Vitamins: Vitamin A 137µg, Vitamin B6 1.3mg, Vitamin C 26mg, Vitamin K 125µg,

Minerals: Niacin 14mg, Phosphorus 420mg, Selenium 46µg, Zinc 3mg

Sugars: 24g

49.   Fish Stew

A great alternative to every day beef stew; fish stew is packed with the traditional vitamins and minerals but with the addition of healthy fats and Omega 3s complete this dish.

Ingredients:

- 1 teaspoon olive oil
- 1 medium green bell pepper, chopped
- 1 medium carrot, chopped
- 1/2 medium onion, chopped
- 1 (14 ounce) can diced tomatoes
- 1 cup water
- 1 Idaho potato, peeled, diced
- 1 teaspoon Cajun seasoning
- 3 (4 ounce) filets halibut, diced

How to Prepare:

In large soup pot, heat the oil over medium-high heat. Cook the bell pepper, carrot, and onion until the onion is soft, stirring frequently. Stir in the tomatoes, water, potato, and Cajun seasoning. Bring to a boil. Reduce the heat and simmer, covered, for 20 minutes, or until the potato pieces are tender.

Gently stir in the fish. Cook, covered, for 5 minutes, or until the fish flakes easily when tested with a fork. Remove from the heat. Ladle into bowls and serve.

Nutritional Information:

Total calories: 589

Vitamins: Vitamin B6 0.5mg, Vitamin E 3mg, Vitamin K 50µg

Minerals: Magnesium 132mg, Phosphorus 433mg, Selenium 85µg, Zinc 4mg

Sugars: 6g

50. Mediterranean Snapper with Cucumber Salad

A spin on the popular Mediterranean diet, this fish dish is a fresh dish overflowing with flavor. Popular Mediterranean spices, such as garlic and cucumber, provide extra nutrients to improve heart function.

Ingredients:

- 4 (4 ounce) red snapper fillets
- 2 tablespoons lemon juice
- 1/2 teaspoon dried oregano
- 1/4 teaspoon paprika
- 1/2 cup salsa
- 3/4 cup cucumber, chopped
- 2 tablespoons capers, drained
- 1/2 teaspoon grated lemon zest
- 1 tablespoon olive oil

How to Prepare:

Preheat the oven to 400 degrees. Lightly spray a 13 x 9 x 2-inch baking pan with nonstick spray.

Arrange the fish in a single layer in the pan. Spoon 2 tablespoons lemon juice over the fish. Sprinkle with the oregano, and paprika.

Bake for 10 minutes, or until the fish flakes easily when tested with a fork. Transfer fish to plates

In a small bowl, combine remaining ingredients. Spoon over fish and serve.

Nutritional Information:

Total calories: 317

Vitamins: Vitamin A 337µg, Vitamin B6 0.3mg, Vitamin C 37mg

Minerals: Phosphorus 207mg, Magnesium 6Mg, Thiamin 0.4mg

Sugars: 6g

51.   Chicken Blueberry Salad

Also known as a superfood, blueberries are loaded with antioxidants which ensure a healthy heart and protects blood vessels

Ingredients

- 5 cups mixed greens
- 1 ½ cup blueberries, divided
- 1/4 cup slivered almonds
- 2 cups cubed chicken breasts, cooked
- 1/4 cup olive oil
- 1/4 cup apple cider vinegar
- 2 tablespoons honey

How to Prepare:

In a large bowl, toss the greens, 1 cup blueberries, almonds, and chicken breasts until well mixed.

In a blender, combine the olive oil, apple cider vinegar, remaining blueberries, and honey. Blend until smooth. Drizzle a few tablespoons over salad and toss to coat.

Serve.

Nutritional Information:

Total calories: 589

Vitamins: Vitamin B6 0.5mg, Vitamin E 3mg, Vitamin K 50µg

Minerals: Magnesium 132mg, Phosphorus 433mg, Selenium 85µg, Zinc 4mg

Sugars: 6g

52. Flank Steak with Avocado Mango Salsa

Together avocado and mango great the perfect paring with beef. This entrée includes iron, healthy fats, and vitamin C to give the heart the boost it needs to function efficiently.

Ingredients

- 2 pounds' flank steak
- 3 tablespoons olive oil
- 3 tablespoons fresh lime juice, divided
- 1 tablespoon Hoisin sauce
- 3 cloves garlic, minced
- 3 oranges, peeled and chopped
- 2 ripe avocados, pitted and chopped
- 1 shallot, minced
- 3 tablespoons chopped fresh parsley

How to Prepare:

Place flank steak in a large zip-lock plastic freezer bag.

Combine oil, 2 tablespoons lime juice, Hoisin, and garlic in a small bowl. Pour over steak; seal and turn to coat.

Refrigerate 1 hour.

Preheat grill or heat a grill pan over medium-high heat. Remove steak from bag, and discard marinade. Grill steak 6 to 7 minutes on each side or until desired degree of doneness. Let stand 10 minutes before slicing.

Meanwhile, combine oranges, avocadoes, shallot, parsley and remaining 1 tablespoon lime juice in a medium bowl.

Serve orange-avocado topping over steak.

Nutritional Information:

Total calories: 416

Vitamins: Vitamin B6 1.4mg, Vitamin B12 2.8µg

Minerals: Phosphorus 559mg, Niacin 23mg

Sugars: 7g

53.   Spicy Tuna with Szechuan Vegetables

A great alternative to salmon, Ahi tuna is packed with B Vitamins. The nutrients found in this fish allow for optimal oxygen circulation and the spicy Szechuan vegetables give the entrée and extra punch.

Ingredients:

- 1 (8 ounce) Ahi Tuna filets

- 3 tablespoons Hoisin sauce

- 2 tablespoons toasted sesame oil

- 2 tablespoons apple cider vinegar

- 1 clove garlic, minced

- 1 teaspoon freshly grated ginger

- 1/4 teaspoon red pepper flakes

- 1 pound fresh green beans, trimmed

- 1 red bell pepper, sliced

- 1 small red onion, sliced

- 2 tablespoons Szechuan sauce

How to Prepare:

Combine 1 tablespoon Hoisin, 2 tablespoons oil, vinegar, garlic and ginger. In a small bowl. Lay tuna in a shallow baking dish and pour the marinade over top. Refrigerate for 30 minutes, or up to 24 hours.

Preheat grill to medium high heat. Grill tuna until firm but still slightly pink inside

Bring pot of water to a boil and add the green beans. Cook for 2 minutes, drain and rinse with ice cold water.

Heat a large skillet or wok over medium high heat. Add remaining sesame oil, followed by the green beans, red peppers and onions. Add remain hoisin sauce and Szechuan sauce and stir quickly for about 1 minute. Serve over Tuna.

Nutritional Information:

Total calories: 441

Vitamins: Vitamin A 216µg, Vitamin B6 1.2mg, Vitamin C 82mg, Vitamin K 183µg

Minerals: Niacin 14mg, Magnesium 115mg, Phosphorus 397mg, Selenium 32µg

Sugars: 9g

54.   Southwest Stuffed Potatoes

Beta-carotene rich potatoes combined with the perfect protein of black beans, make this   stuffed   potato   a powerhouse. This will keep your heart pumping and strong

Ingredients:

- 3 medium Russet potatoes, scrubbed
- 1 tablespoon olive oil
- 1 (15 ounce) can fire roasted tomatoes, with juices
- 1 cup black beans, cooked
- 1 teaspoon ground cumin
- 1 teaspoon chili powder
- 1/2 teaspoon garlic powder
- 1/2 cup shredded cheddar cheese
- 3 green onions, sliced

How to Prepare:

Preheat oven to 400 degrees.

Pierce the potatoes with a fork, rub with oil and bake for 45-50 minutes, until tender.

Meanwhile, mix the tomatoes, black beans and seasonings in a medium bowl.

When the potatoes are done, slice in half lengthwise. Scoop out most of the potato and add to the bowl with the bean mixture. Mix and divide between the potato shells. Top with cheese and return to the oven. Bake for 10-15 minutes, or until cheese is melted. Top with green onion and serve.

Nutritional Information:

Total calories: 518

Vitamins: Vitamin A 137µg, Vitamin B6 1.3mg, Vitamin C 26mg, Vitamin K 125µg,

Minerals: Niacin 14mg, Phosphorus 420mg, Selenium 46µg, Zinc 3mg

Sugars: 24g

55.   Honey Mustard Chicken Skewers

A year round summer dish, these skewers can be grilled or baked. When grilled, these skewers have a wonderful smoky sweet flavor and excess Vitamin A!

Ingredients:

- 1 pound boneless, skinless chicken breasts, cubed
- 1 red pepper, cubed
- 1 red onion, cubed
- 10 grape tomatoes
- 3 tablespoons olive oil
- 1 tablespoon Dijon mustard
- 2 tablespoons honey
- 1 cup Couscous

How to Prepare:

Preheat oven to 375 degrees. Line a baking sheet with foil and spray with nonstick spray.

Skewer chicken, pepper, onion, and tomato onto skewers, alternating items until none remain.

In small bowl, combine remaining ingredients. Brush over skewers and place onto prepared pan.

Bake for about 25 to 30 minutes, until cooked through. Serve Over couscous.

Nutritional Information:

Total calories: 532

Vitamins: Vitamin A 413µg, B-6 0.6mg, B-12 1.4µg, Vitamin C 76mg, Vitamin K 300µg

Minerals: Copper 850 µg, Iron 4mg, Magnesium 97mg, Niacin 9mg, Phosphorus 599mg, Selenium 46µg, Zinc 4mg

Sugars 12g

56. Slow Cooker Southwest Chili

A quick dish for a winter's night, the chilling will keep you warm and your heart pumping. Packed with iron and protein, this keeps blood vessels strong and open for essential circulation.

Ingredients:

- 1-pound lean ground turkey, ground and cooked
- 1 cup kidney beans
- 1 clove garlic, minced
- 1/2 cup onion, chopped
- 3 cups chicken bone broth
- 1 1/2 cups corn kernels
- 1/2 cup red pepper, diced
- 2 tablespoons chili powder
- 1 teaspoon cumin

How to Prepare:

Add all remaining ingredients to the slow cooker and cook on low for 6 to 8 hours or high for 4. Serve.

Nutritional Information:

Total calories: 310

Vitamins: Vitamin D 9µg, Vitamin E 4mg, Vitamin K 62µg

Minerals: Phosphorus 223mg, Selenium 21µg, Niacin 5mg

Sugars 6g

57.   Balsamic Spinach and Vegetable Wrap

Balsamic vinegar gives these veggies wrap a little zip to create a wonderful light and quick meal. Packed with several different vegetables, this wrap contains a variety of vitamin and minerals to help with everyday heart function.

Ingredients:

- 1 tablespoon olive oil
- 1 small zucchini, cut into thin strips
- 1 red bell pepper, cut into thin strips
- 1 small onion, cut into thin strips
- 1/4 cup mushrooms, chopped
- 1/2 cup spinach
- 2 clove garlic, minced
- 2 tablespoon honey
- 1/4 cup balsamic vinegar
- 2 large whole wheat tortillas

How to prepare:

In medium skillet, heat olive oil on medium heat. Once hot,

combine all ingredients with exception of honey, vinegar, and tortillas. Cook until veggies are soft.

In small sauce pan, combine honey and vinegar. Cook on medium heat, bring to a boil and simmer until slightly thickened. Stir frequently.

On flat surface, lay tortillas. Divide cooked veggies between the tortillas and drizzle vinegar and honey sauce over the top. Fold in the sides and roll into a burrito shape. Serve.

Nutritional Information:

Total calories: 522

Vitamins: Vitamin A 284µg, Vitamin B6 0.6mg, Vitamin C 99mg, Vitamin K 190µg

Minerals: Potassium 1047mg, Phosphorus 283mg

Sugars: 44g

58.   Halibut with Chickpeas and Tomato

Tomato is a great source of Vitamin C and can easily be added to any dish. Try tomato with chickpea and halibut for a change, to try something new, or just for a vitamin C boost.

Ingredients:

- 2 tablespoons olive oil

- 1 green onion, finely chopped

- 8 cherry tomatoes, quartered

- 4 fresh sage leaves, chopped

- 1 cup chickpeas

- 2 (6 ounce) halibut filets

How to Prepare:

Over medium heat, in a saucepan add half the oil and onion. Cook green onion until translucent. Add the tomatoes, sage, and chickpeas. Turn off the heat and cover to keep warm.

Over medium to high heat, in a separate saucepan with remaining oil, brown both sides of the fish. Fish is cooked through when firm and flaky.

To serve, transfer the chickpeas to the serving plate. Put the fish on top. Serve

Nutritional Information:

Total calories: 229

Vitamins: Vitamin A 178µg, Vitamin B6 0.4mg, Vitamin B12 1.5µg, Vitamin C 26mg, Vitamin K 113µg

Minerals: Phosphorus 365mg, Selenium 54µg, Magnesium 32mg

Sugars 4g

59.   Lasagna Rolls

This lasagna entree full of vitamins and minerals to keep your heart active. Each roll is the perfect serving size for an individual dinner or an addition to a family meal.

Ingredients:

- 10 whole wheat lasagna noodles, cooked
- 1 (24 ounce) jar marinara sauce
- 1 tablespoon olive oil
- 2 cloves garlic, minced
- 6 cups baby spinach, chopped
- 1 cup ricotta cheese
- 1 1/2 shredded mozzarella
- 1/2 cup cottage cheese (small curd if possible)
- 1 egg white
- 1 teaspoon dried oregano
- 1/4 cup grated parmesan cheese

How to Prepare:

Preheat oven to 425 degrees. Add 1 1/4 cups marinara to a

13" x 9" x 2" casserole dish.

In a large skillet, add oil and heat to medium-low heat. Sauté garlic until fragrant, about 1 minute. Add chopped spinach and sauté until wilted, about 3 minutes.

In a large mixing bowl, combine garlic, spinach, ricotta, 1 cup mozzarella, cottage cheese, egg white, oregano, salt and pepper.

On a work surface, lined with parchment paper, arrange lasagna noodles flat, add 1/4 cup cheese and spinach mixture to each noodle, spread evenly to cover noodles. Start rolling the noodle at the end closest to you. Place lasagna rolls seam side down, not quite touching, in the prepared casserole dish. Evenly spread 1 cup marinara over rolls, sprinkle with remaining mozzarella and parmesan.

Cover with aluminum foil and bake 20 minutes, or until cheese is hot and bubbly. If desired, serve rolls with additional heated marinara.

Nutritional Information:

Total calories: 518

Vitamins: Vitamin A 137µg, Vitamin B6 1.3mg, Vitamin C 26mg, Vitamin K 125µg,

Minerals: Niacin 14mg, Phosphorus 420mg, Selenium 46µg, Zinc 3mg

Sugars: 24g

60. Roasted Citrus Beet Salad

Sweet honey and orange citrus make this beet salad a wonderful earthy salad. Beets contain a high level of nitrates, which widen blood vessels and allow an increased blood flow to the heart and body.

Ingredients:

- 2 red beets, peeled and diced large
- 2 golden beets, peeled and diced large
- 2 tablespoons olive oil
- 1 tablespoon fresh rosemary, chopped
- 1 tablespoon orange zest
- 3 cups spinach
- 1 large orange, peeled and cut into wedges
- 1/4 cup walnuts
- 1/4 cup crumbled soft goat cheese
- 2 tablespoons honey
- 2 tablespoons balsamic vinegar

How to prepare:

Preheat oven to 450 degrees.

Toss both beets in olive oil, rosemary, and orange zest. Bake for 20 to 25 minutes, stirring every 10 minutes. Bake until soft. Remove from oven and cool completely.

In large bowl, toss cooked beets, spinach, oranges, walnuts and cheese. Divide into serving bowls. Drizzle with honey and vinegar to serve.

Nutritional Information:

Total calories: 473

Vitamins: Vitamin A 292μg, Vitamin C 56mg, Vitamin K 238μg

Minerals: Magnesium 114mg, Phosphorus 232mg

Sugars: 38g

61.   Broccolini Pasta with Parmesan

If you like broccoli, you'll love broccolini! A hybrid of broccoli and kale, broccolini contains the nutrients of each vegetable. Giving it a healthy dose of Vitamins C and K – essential for proper heart function.

Ingredients:

- 1 tablespoon olive oil

- 2 cups Broccolini, chopped

- 2 clove garlic, minced

- 1/2-pound whole wheat linguini, cooked

- 2 tablespoons basil pesto

- 1/2 cup shredded parmesan

How to prepare:

In skillet, heat olive oil on medium heat. Add Broccolini and garlic. Cook until Broccolini is bright green and just beginning to soften. Add linguini and cook until hot. Stir in pesto and 3/4 of the parmesan. Spoon into bowls and top with remaining parmesan. Serve.

Nutritional Information:

Total calories: 332

Vitamins: Vitamin C 40mg, Vitamin K 56 µg

Minerals: Phosphorus 266mg, Selenium 45µg

Sugars: 2g

62. Rye and Arugula Poach Egg Sandwich

Creamy, crunchy, and packed with vitamins and minerals! Rye is highly nutritious, giving the heart a boost of magnesium – which prevents loss of heart function.

Ingredients:

- 1/4 cup feta cheese
- 2 tablespoons grated parmesan cheese
- 1/4 teaspoon dried thyme
- 1 tablespoon lemon juice, divided
- 3 cups water
- 2 tablespoons apple cider vinegar
- 2 eggs
- 1 cup arugula
- 1/4 teaspoon cayenne pepper

How to prepare:

Crumble the feta and mix with the Parmesan, thyme and half the lemon juice.

Toss the arugula and bean sprouts with oil and remaining

lemon juice.

Bring water and vinegar to boil in medium sauce pot. Reduce to a simmer and swirl water to create movement. While water continues to move, crack eggs one at a time into the water. Remove from heat and let sit for 5 to 8 minutes depend on doneness of yolk preference.

One each slice of rye bread, evenly top with arugula and bean sprouts. Followed by feta mix. With a slotted spoon, remove egg from water and place on top of feta. Sprinkle with cayenne and serve.

Nutritional Information:

Total calories: 212

Vitamins: Vitamin B12 0.9mg

Minerals: Phosphorus 232mg, Selenium 28 µg, Riboflavin 0.5mg

Sugars: 2g

JUICES

1.   Carrot Apple Juice

Ingredients:

2 large carrots

1 large Honeycrisp apple, cored

2 large kiwis, peeled

1 cup of mint, chopped

1 large orange, peeled

2 oz of water

Preparation:

Wash the carrots and cut into thick slices. Set aside

Wash the apple and remove the core. Cut into bite-sized pieces and set aside.

Peel the kiwis and cut lengthwise in half. Set aside.

Wash the fresh mint and roughly chop it. Set aside.

Now, combine kiwis, carrots, apple, and mint in a juicer and process until juiced. Transfer to serving glasses and add some ice before serving.

Enjoy!

Nutritional information per serving: Kcal: 292, Protein: 6.1g, Carbs: 88.6g, Fats: 1.8g

2.   Cabbage Lemon Juice

Ingredients:

1 cup of purple cabbage, torn

1 large lemon, peeled

2 cups of Brussels sprouts

2 cups of fennel

1 cup of beet greens, torn

1 large cucumber

Preparation:

Combine cabbage and beet greens in a colander and wash under cold running water. Torn with hands and set aside.

Wash the Brussels sprouts and trim off the outer leaves. Cut in half and set aside.

Wash the fennel bulb and trim off the wilted outer layers. Cut into small chunks and set aside.

Wash the cucumber and cut into thick slices. Set aside.

Now, combine Brussels sprouts, fennel, cabbage, beet

greens, and cucumber in a juicer and process until juiced.

Transfer to serving glasses and add few ice cubes before serving.

Enjoy!

Nutritional information per serving: Kcal: 154, Protein: 12.8g, Carbs: 53g, Fats: 1.5g

3.　　Zucchini Pomegranate Juice

Ingredients:

1 large zucchini, seeded

1 cup of pomegranate seeds

1 large orange, peeled

3 large kiwis, peeled

1 large lime, peeled

Preparation:

Wash the zucchini and cut in half. Scoop out the seeds using a spoon. Cut into small chunks and set aside.

Cut the top of the pomegranate fruit using a sharp knife. Slice down to each of the white membranes inside of the fruit. Pop the seeds into a measuring cup and set aside.

Peel the orange and divide into wedges. Set aside.

Peel the kiwis and cut lengthwise in half. Set aside.

Peel the lime and cut lengthwise in half. Set aside.

Now, process kiwis, zucchini, lime, pomegranate seeds,

and orange in a juicer.

Transfer to a serving glasses and add some ice cubes before serving.

Nutritional information per serving: Kcal: 183, Protein: 8.5g, Carbs: 52.6g, Fats: 1.6g

4. Mango Banana Juice

Ingredients:

1 cup of mango, chunked

1 large banana, sliced

1 large carrot, sliced

1 whole lime, peeled

1 small Golden Delicious apple, cored

¼ tsp of cinnamon, ground

Preparation:

Peel the mango and cut into small chunks. Fill the measuring cup and reserve the rest in the refrigerator. Set aside.

Peel the banana and cut into slices. Set aside.

Wash and peel the carrot. Cut into thin slices and set aside.

Peel the lime and cut lengthwise in half. Set aside.

Wash the apple and cut in half. Remove the core and chop into bite-sized pieces. Set aside.

Now, combine carrot, lime, mango, banana, and apple in a juicer and process until juiced. Transfer to a serving glass and stir in the cinnamon.

Add some ice and serve immediately.

Nutrition information per serving: Kcal: 290, Protein: 4.1g, Carbs: 83.9g, Fats: 1.5g

5.   Kale Asparagus Juice

Ingredients:

1 cup of kale, chopped

1 cup of asparagus, trimmed

1 large fennel bulb

1 large artichoke head

1 cup of Brussel sprouts, trimmed

1 cup of Swiss chard, chopped

¼ tsp of Cayenne pepper, ground

Preparation:

Combine kale and Swiss chard in a colander and wash under cold running water. Roughly chop it and set aside.

Wash the asparagus and trim off the woody ends. Cut into small pieces and set aside.

Wash the fennel bulb and trim off the wilted outer layers. Cut into small chunks and set aside.

Trim off the outer leaves of the artichoke. Wash it and cut

into bite-sized pieces. Set aside.

Wash the Brussel sprouts and trim off the outer layers. Cut in half and set aside.

Now, process fennel, artichoke, kale, asparagus, Brussel sprouts, and Swiss chard in a juicer. Transfer to serving glasses and stir in the Cayenne pepper.

Refrigerate for 10 minutes before serving.

Nutritional information per serving: Kcal: 154, Protein: 17.6g, Carbs: 54.4g, Fats: 1.8g

6.   Orange Mint Juice

Ingredients:

1 large orange

2 cups of fresh mint, torn

2 cups of fresh raspberries

1 large green apple, cored

1 large lime

2 oz of water

Preparation:

Peel the orange and divide into wedges. Set aside.

Wash the mint thoroughly and torn with hands. Set aside. Wash the raspberries under cold running water and set aside.

Peel the apple and remove the core. Cut into bite-sized pieces and set aside. Peel the lime and cut lengthwise in half. Set aside.

Now, process raspberries, mint, orange, apple, and lime in a juicer. Transfer to serving glasses and stir in the water.

Add some ice and serve immediately.

Nutritional information per serving: Kcal: 258, Protein: 7.6g, Carbs: 90.1g, Fats: 2.7g

7.   Lemon Honey Juice

Ingredients:

1 large lemon, peeled

1 tbsp of liquid honey

1 cup of blueberries

1 large orange, peeled

1 large green apple, cored

Preparation:

Peel the lemon and cut lengthwise in half. Set aside.

Place the blueberries in a colander and wash under cold running water. Drain and set aside.

Peel the orange and divide into wedges. Set aside.

Wash the apple and remove the core. Cut into bite-sized pieces and set aside. Now, combine blueberries, lemon, orange, and apple in a juicer and process until juiced. Transfer to serving glasses and stir in the liquid honey.

Add few ice cubes or refrigerate before serving

Nutritional information per serving: Kcal: 305, Protein: 4.3g, Carbs: 76.5g, Fats: 1.3g

8.   Grapefruit Lime Juice

Ingredients:

2 large grapefruits

1 large lime

2 cups of celery, chopped

2 large carrots

1 ginger root slice, 1-inch

2 oz of water

Preparation:

Peel the grapefruits and divide into wedges. Set aside.

Peel the lime lengthwise in half. Set aside.

Wash the celery and chop into small pieces. About 2 large stalks will be enough. Set aside.

Wash the carrots and cut into thick slices. Set aside.

Peel the ginger slice and set aside.

Now, process celery, grapefruits, lime, carrots, and ginger in a juicer. Transfer to serving glasses and stir in the water.

Refrigerate for 15 minutes before serving.

Enjoy!

Nutritional information per serving: Kcal: 250, Protein: 6.7g, Carbs: 76.3g, Fats: 1.4g

9.   Kiwi Celery Juice

Ingredients:

1 large kiwi, peeled

3 celery stalks

½ medium-sized grapefruit, peeled

1 large lemon, peeled

¼ tsp of ginger, ground

¼ tsp of Cayenne pepper, ground

A handful of watercress

Preparation:

Peel the kiwi and cut into halves. Set aside.

Wash the grapefruit and cut into halves. Chop one half into small cubes and reserve the other half for later. Set aside.

Peel the lemon and cut into quarters. Set aside.

Wash the watercress in and roughly chop it.

Now, process kiwi, grapefruit, lemon, and celery in a juicer until juiced.

Transfer to serving glasses and stir in the Cayenne pepper and ginger. You can add a pinch of Himalayan salt, but this is optional.

Serve immediately.

Nutritional information per serving: Kcal: 61, Protein: 2.1g, Carbs: 20.4g, Fats: 1.1g

10.   Cinnamon Mango Juice

Ingredients:

1 cup of mango, chunked

1 large peach, pitted

1 medium-sized Granny Smith's apple, cored

1 whole lemon, peeled

¼ tsp of cinnamon, ground

Preparation:

Peel the mango and cut into small chunks. Fill the measuring cup and reserve the rest in the refrigerator. Set aside.

Wash the peach and cut in half. Remove the pit and chop into small pieces. Set aside.

Wash the apple and cut lengthwise in half. Remove the core and chop into bite-sized pieces. Set aside.

Peel the lemon and cut lengthwise in half. Set aside.

Now, combine peach, apple, lemon, and mango in a juicer and process until juiced. Transfer to a serving glass and stir in the cinnamon.

Add some crushed ice and serve immediately.

Enjoy!

Nutrition information per serving: Kcal: 236, Protein: 4.3g, Carbs: 69.5g, Fats: 1.5g

11.   Apple Kale Juice

Ingredients:

1 large green apple, cored

1 cup of fresh kale

3 large kiwis

1 large lemon

1 cup of fresh mint

A handful of fresh spinach

3 oz of water

Preparation:

Wash the apple and remove the core. Cut into bite-sized pieces and set aside.

Wash kale, mint, and spinach and combine in a large bowl. Pour hot water enough to cover the ingredients. Let it soak for 10 minutes. Drain and torn with hands. Set aside.

Peel the kiwis and lemon. Cut lengthwise in half and set aside.

Now, process kiwis, lemon, kale, mint, spinach, and apple in a juicer. Transfer to serving glasses and stir in the water.

Add some ice and serve immediately.

Enjoy!

Nutritional information per serving: Kcal: 246, Protein: 8.6g, Carbs: 74.5g, Fats: 2.6g

12.   Sweet Beet Juice

Ingredients:

1 cup of beets, trimmed and chopped

3 large carrots

1 large cucumber

1 large orange, peeled

2 oz of water

½ tsp of agave nectar

Preparation:

Wash the beets and trim off the green parts. Cut into bite-sized pieces and fill the measuring cup. Reserve the rest for some other juice.

Wash the carrots and cut into thick slices. Set aside.

Wash the cucumber and cut into thick slices. Set aside.

Peel the orange and divide into wedges. Set aside.

Now, combine carrots, beets, cucumber, and orange in a juicer and process until juiced.

Transfer to serving glasses and stir in the water and agave nectar. Add some ice and serve immediately.

Nutritional information per serving: Kcal: 296, Protein: 7.9g, Carbs: 86.2g, Fats: 1.3g

13.   Cantaloupe Orange Juice

Ingredients:

2 cups of blackberries

1 cup of cantaloupe, diced

1 large orange

1 large lemon

1 small Granny Smith's apple

Preparation:

Cut the cantaloupe in half. Scoop out the seeds and flesh. Cut two wedges and peel them. Chop into chunks and set aside. Reserve the rest of the cantaloupe in a refrigerator.

Peel the orange and divide into wedges. Set aside.

Place the blackberries in a colander and wash under cold running water. Drain and set aside.

Peel the lemon and cut lengthwise in half. Set aside.

Wash the apple and remove the core. Cut into bite-sized pieces and set aside.

Now, combine blackberries, cantaloupe, orange, lemon, and apple in a juicer and process until juiced. Transfer to serving glasses and refrigerate for 10 minutes before serving.

Enjoy!

Nutritional information per serving: Kcal: 258, Protein: 8.3g, Carbs: 87g, Fats: 2.4g

14.   Tomato Lemon Juice

Ingredients:

1 cup of cherry tomatoes, halved

1 large lemon, peeled

1 cup of basil, torn

1 large red bell pepper, seeded

1 rosemary sprig

¼ tsp of Himalayan salt

Preparation:

Wash the tomatoes and place in a bowl. Cut in half and reserve the juice while cutting. Set aside.

Peel the lemon and cut lengthwise in half. Set aside.

Wash the basil thoroughly under cold running water using acolander. Drain and torn with hands. Set aside.

Wash the bell pepper and cut in half. Remove the seeds and cut into small pieces. Set aside.

Now, combine tomatoes, basil, pepper, and lemon in a

juicer and process until juiced. Transfer to serving glasses and stir in the salt. Sprinkle with some rosemary for some extra taste.

Refrigerate for 10 minutes before serving.

Nutritional information per serving: Kcal: 189, Protein: 19.5g, Carbs: 53.1g, Fats: 2.6g

15.   Garlic Kale Juice

Ingredients:

4 fresh kale leaves

1 garlic clove, peeled

2 large oranges, peeled

½ cup of fresh broccoli, chopped

3 large carrots

4 collard green leaves

¼ tsp of Himalayan salt

2 oz of water

Preparation:

Combine collard greens and kale in a colander and wash under cold running water. Roughly chop and set aside.

Peel the garlic clove and set aside.

Peel the oranges and divide into wedges. Set aside.

Wash the broccoli and chop into small pieces. set aside.

Wash the carrots and cut into small pieces. set aside.

Process oranges, broccoli, carrots, collard greens, kale and garlic in a juicer. Transfer to serving glasses and stir in the Himalayan salt and water.

Serve immediately.

Nutritional information per serving: Kcal: 171, Protein: 9.2g, Carbs: 43.3g, Fats: 2.3g

16.   Artichoke Zucchini Juice

Ingredients:

1 medium-sized artichoke, chopped

1 small zucchini, sliced

1 cup of sweet potatoes, cubed

1 whole lime, peeled

1 large carrot, sliced

¼ tsp of salt

¼ tsp of turmeric, ground

Preparation:

Wash the artichoke and trim off the outer leaves. Cut into small pieces and fill the measuring cup. Reserve the rest in the refrigerator.

Peel the zucchini and cut into thin slices. Set aside.

Peel the potatoes and cut into small cubes. Place in a deep pot and add 3 cups of water. Bring it to a boil and cook for 5 minutes. Remove from the heat and drain well. Set aside to cool completely.

Peel the lime and cut lengthwise in half. Set aside.

Wash and peel the carrot. Cut into thin slices and set aside.

Now, combine potatoes, artichoke, zucchini, lime, and carrots in a juicer and process until juiced. Transfer to a serving glass and stir in the salt and turmeric.

Refrigerate for 10 minutes before serving.

Nutrition information per serving: Kcal: 177, Protein: 8.6g, Carbs: 54.5g, Fats: 0.8g

17.   Watermelon Kiwi Juice

Ingredients:

1 cup of watermelon

1 large kiwi

1 large orange

1 large green apple, cored

1 large guava

3 oz of coconut water

Preparation:

Cut the watermelon lengthwise. For one cup, you will need about one large wedge. Peel and cut into chunks. Remove the seeds and set aside. Reserve the rest of the melon for some other juices.

Peel the kiwi and cut lengthwise in half. Set aside.

Wash the guava and cut into chunks. If you are using large fruit, reserve the rest for some other recipe in a refrigerator.

Peel the orange and divide into wedges. Set aside.

Wash the apple and remove the core. Cut into bite-sized pieces and set aside.

Now, combine guava, watermelon, orange, kiwi, and apple in a juicer and process until juiced. Transfer to serving glasses and stir in the coconut water.

Add some ice or refrigerate before serving.

Enjoy!

Nutritional information per serving: Kcal: 264, Protein: 5.6g, Carbs: 73.8g, Fats: 1.6g

18. Cherry Vanilla Juice

Ingredients:

1 cup of cherries, pitted

1 cup of cranberries

3 whole apricots, pitted and chopped

1 small Golden Delicious apple, cored

1 tsp of vanilla extract

3 tbsp of coconut water

Preparation:

Rinse the cherries under cold running water. Drain and cut each cherry in half. Remove the pits and set aside.

Rinse the cranberries using a large colander. Drain and set aside.

Wash the apricots and cut in half. Remove the pits and chop into small pieces. Set aside.

Wash the apple and cut lengthwise in half. Remove the core and chop into small pieces. Set aside.

Now, combine cranberries, apricots, apple, and cherries in a juicer and process until juiced. Transfer to a serving glass and stir in the vanilla extract and coconut water.

Sprinkle with some finely chopped mint for some extra taste. However, it's optional.

Add few ice cubes and serve immediately.

Nutrition information per serving: Kcal: 216, Protein: 3.8g, Carbs: 66.1g, Fats: 1.1g

19.   Apple Carrot Juice

Ingredients:

2 large apples, cored

2 large carrots

½ cup of fresh spinach

¼ tsp of ginger, ground

2 tbsp of fresh parsley

1 tbsp of flaxseeds

Preparation:

Wash the apples and remove the core. Cut into bite-sized pieces and set aside.

Wash and chop the carrots into small pieces. Set aside.

Wash the spinach thoroughly under cold running water. Drain and torn into small pieces. Set aside.

Now, process all in a juicer until well juiced. Transfer to serving glasses and stir in the ginger. Sprinkle with flaxseeds for some extra nutrients and serve immediately!

Nutritional information per serving: Kcal: 119, Protein: 4.3g, Carbs: 62.2g, Fats: 2.3g

20.   Lemon Ginger Juice

Ingredients:

1 large lemon, peeled

½ tsp of ginger, ground

½ cup of cilantro

3 celery stalks

1 large green apple, cored

Preparation:

Peel the lemon and cut into quarters. Process in a juicer until juiced.

Wash the cilantro and chop it roughly. Set aside.

Wash the celery stalks and chop into small pieces. Set aside.

Wash the apple and remove the core. Cut into bite-sized pieces and set aside. Now, process cilantro, celery, and apple. Transfer to serving glasses and stir in the ginger. Refrigerate for 15 minutes or add some ice before serving.

Enjoy!

Nutritional information per serving: Kcal: 73, Protein: 2.2g, Carbs: 26.7g, Fats: 0.1g

21. Pumpkin Lettuce Juice

Ingredients:

1 cup of yellow pumpkin, chopped

1 cup of Romaine lettuce, chopped

2 large leeks, chopped

1 cup of asparagus, trimmed

2 tbsp of fresh parsley, chopped

1 large cucumber

Preparation:

Peel the pumpkin and cut in half. Scoop out the seeds using a spoon. Cut one large wedge and peel it. Cut into small chunks and fill the measuring cup. Reserve the rest for some other juice.

Combine lettuce and parsley in a colander and wash thoroughly under cold running water. Drain and roughly chop it.

Wash the leeks and chop into small pieces. Set aside.

Wash the asparagus and trim off the woody ends. Chop

into small pieces and set aside.

Wash the cucumber and cut into thick slices. Set aside.

Now, process leeks, asparagus, pumpkin, lettuce, parsley, and cucumber in a juicer. Transfer to serving glasses and add some ice, or refrigerate for 20 minutes before serving.

Nutritional information per serving: Kcal: 185, Protein: 9.5g, Carbs: 50.8g, Fats: 1.3g

22.   Broccoli Lemon Juice

Ingredients:

1 cup of fennel, chopped

1 cup of spinach, torn

1 cup of broccoli, chopped

1 whole lemon, peeled

1 whole lime, peeled

¼ tsp of ginger, ground

Preparation:

Wash the broccoli and trim off the outer leaves. Chop into small pieces and fill the measuring cup. Reserve the rest in the refrigerator.

Peel the lemon and lime. Cut lengthwise into halves. Set aside.

Trim off the fennel stalks and outer wilted layers. Wash and chop the fennel into bite-sized pieces. Fill the measuring cup and reserve the rest for later. Set aside.

Rinse the spinach thoroughly under cold running water and

drain. Torn into small piecesand set aside.

Now, combine fennel, spinach, broccoli, lemon, and lime in a juicer. Process until juiced.

Transfer to a serving glass and stir in the ginger.

Add some crushed ice and serve immediately.

Nutrition information per serving: Kcal: 86, Protein: 10.5g, Carbs: 29.1g, Fats: 1.5g

23. Kale Artichoke Juice

Ingredients:

1 cup of kale, chopped

1 medium-sized artichoke head

3 cups of beet greens

1 bunch of spinach

1 large cucumber

3 tbsp of parsley, chopped

¼ tsp of Himalayan salt

Preparation:

Combine beet greens, spinach, kale and parsley in a large colander. Wash thoroughly under cold running water. Drain and roughly chop it. Set aside.

Trim off the outer wilted layers of the artichoke. Wash and cut into small pieces. Set aside.

Wash the cucumber and cut into thick slices. Set aside.

Now, combine beet greens, spinach, kale, artichoke,

cucumber, and parsley in a juicer and process until juiced.

Transfer to serving glasses and stir in the salt.

Add some ice and serve immediately.

Nutritional information per serving: Kcal: 151, Protein: 21.6g, Carbs: 48.2g, Fats: 2.7g

24.   Apple Cinnamon Juice

Ingredients:

1 small Golden Delicious apple, chopped

1 medium-sized orange, peeled

1 medium-sized pear, chopped

1 cup of beets, chopped

¼ tsp of cinnamon, ground

¼ tsp of ginger, ground

Preparation:

Wash the apple and cut lengthwise in half. Remove the core and cut into bite-sized pieces. Set aside.

Peel the orange and divide into wedges. Cut each wedge in half and set aside.

Wash the pear and cut in half. Remove the core and chop into small pieces. Set aside.

Wash the beets and trim off the green ends. Cut into slices and fill the measuring cup. Reserve the rest for later.

Now, combine orange, pear, beets, and apple in a juicer and process until juiced.

Transfer to a serving glass and stir in the cinnamon and ginger. Add some ice before serving.

Enjoy!

Nutrition information per serving: Kcal: 234, Protein: 4.4g, Carbs: 73.1g, Fats: 0.8g

25. Pumpkin Carrot Juice

Ingredients:

1 cup of pumpkin chunks

1 large carrot

1 large yellow apple, cored

1 large orange

¼ tsp of cinnamon, ground

3 oz of water

Preparation:

Peel the pumpkin and cut in half. Scoop out the seeds using a spoon. Cut one large wedge and peel it. Cut into small chunks and set aside. Reserve the rest for later.

Wash the carrot and cut into thick slices. Set aside.

Wash the apple and remove the core. Cut into bite-sized pieces and set aside.

Peel the orange and divide into wedges. Set aside.

Now, process pumpkin, apple, carrot, and orange in a

juicer. Transfer to serving glasses and stir in the cinnamon and water.

Add few ice cubes and serve immediately.

Enjoy!

Nutritional information per serving: Kcal: 220, Protein: 4.1g, Carbs: 65.3g, Fats: 0.8g

26. Cantaloupe Pineapple Juice

Ingredients:

1 cup of cantaloupe, peeled

½ pineapple, peeled

2 large green apples, cored

½ cup of fresh kale

Preparation:

Peel and chop the cantaloupe into small cubes. Remove the seeds and set aside.

Peel the pineapple and cut into small chunks. Set aside.

Wash the apples and remove the core. Cut into bite-sized pieces and set aside.

Wash thoroughly the kale and soak in water for 10 minutes. Set aside. Process cantaloupe, apple, pineapple, and kale in a juicer until nicely juiced. Transfer to serving glasses and add some ice before serving. You can add some liquid honey to taste, but this is optional.

Nutritional information per serving: Kcal: 115, Protein: 1.2g, Carbs: 28.8g, Fats: 1.2g

27.   Lime Watercress Juice

Ingredients:

3 large limes, peeled

1 cup of watercress

1 cup of beets, trimmed

1 large green apple, cored

1 large cucumber

Preparation:

Peel the limes and cut lengthwise in half. Set aside.

Wash the watercress thoroughly under cold running water. Drain and set aside.

Wash the beets and trim off the green ends. Cut into bite-sized pieces and set aside.

Wash the apple and remove the core. Cut into bite-sized pieces. Set aside.

Wash the cucumber and cut into thick slices. Set aside.

Now, combine beets, limes, watercress, apple, and

cucumber in a juicer and process until juiced.

Add some ice and serve.

Nutritional information per serving: Kcal: 211, Protein: 6.4g, Carbs: 63.5g, Fats: 1.1g

28. Kiwi Apple Juice

Ingredients:

2 large kiwis, peeled

1 large Fuji apple, cored

2 cups of blueberries

1 cup of watermelon, seeded

2 oz of coconut water

Preparation:

Peel the kiwis and cut lengthwise in half. Set aside.

Wash the apple and remove the core. Cut into bite-sized pieces and set aside.

Wash the blueberries under cold running water using a colander. Drain and set aside.

Cut the watermelon in half. Cut one large wedge and peel it. Chop into small chunks and remove the seeds. Fill the measuring cup and refrigerate the rest for some other juice.

Now, combine blueberries, kiwis, apple, and watermelon in

a juicer and process until juiced. Transfer to serving glasses and stir in coconut water.

Add some ice and serve immediately.

Nutritional information per serving: Kcal: 315, Protein: 7.2g, Carbs: 97.9g, Fats: 2.8g

29.   Beet Celery Juice

Ingredients:

1 cup of beets, sliced

1 cup of celery, cut into bite-sized pieces

1 cup of avocado, cubed

1 whole lemon, peeled

1 oz of water

Preparation:

Wash the beets and trim off the green ends. Slightly peel and cut into thin slices. Fill the measuring cup and reserve the rest for later.

Wash the celery and cut into bite-sized pieces. Fill the measuring cup and reserve the rest in the refrigerator.

Peel the avocado and cut lengthwise in half. Remove the pit and cut into small cubes. Fill the measuring cup and reserve the rest in the refrigerator. Set aside.

Peel the lemon and cut lengthwise in half. Set aside.

Now, combine avocado, beets, celery, and lemon in a

juicer. Process until juiced.

Transfer to a serving glass and stir in the water. Refrigerate for 10 minutes before serving.

Nutrition information per serving: Kcal: 264, Protein: 6.5g, Carbs: 34.2g, Fats: 22.5g

30.   Cherry Mint Juice

Ingredients:

1 cup of cherries, pitted

2 tbsp of fresh mint, chopped

2 cups of green grapes

1 medium-sized Fuji apple, cored

1 tbsp of liquid honey

2 oz of water

Preparation:

Combine grapes and cherries in a large colander. Wash under cold running water and drain. Cut the cherries in half and remove the pits. Set aside.

Wash the mint and roughly chop it. Set aside.

Wash the apple and remove the core. Cut into bite-sized pieces and set aside. Now, combine grapes, cherries, apple, and mint in a juicer and process until juiced. Transfer to serving glasses and add some ice before serving.

Nutritional information per serving: Kcal: 369, Protein: 3.5g, Carbs: 104g, Fats: 1.4g

31.   Grapefruit Kale Juice

Ingredients:

½ cup of grapefruit, chopped

3-4 fresh kale leaves

2 large oranges, peeled

1 tsp of liquid honey

¼ tsp of ginger, ground

Preparation:

Wash the grapefruit and cut into halves. Cut one-half into small pieces. Reserve the other half in a fridge.

Wash the kale leaves and roughly chop it.

Peel the oranges and divide into wedges. Set aside.

Now, process oranges, grapefruit, and kale in a juicer. Transfer to serving glasses and add some water to adjust the thickness if needed.

Stir in the liquid honey and ginger. Add some ice and serve immediately.

Nutritional information per serving: Kcal: 128, Protein: 7.3g, Carbs: 34.5g, Fats: 1.1g

32.   Cucumber Apple Juice

Ingredients:

1 cup of cucumber, sliced

1 medium-sized Golden Delicious apple, cored

1 large banana, peeled

2 whole kiwis, peeled

1 cup of fresh mint, torn

Preparation:

Wash the cucumber and cut into thin slices. Fill the measuring cup and reserve the rest for later. Set aside.

Wash the apple and cut lengthwise in half. Remove the core and cut into bite-sized pieces. Set aside.

Peel the banana and cut into thin slices. Set aside.

Peel the kiwis and cut lengthwise in half. Set aside.

Rinse the mint thoroughly under cold running water and drain. Torn into small pieces and set aside.

Now, combine kiwis, cucumber, apple, and banana in a

juicer and process until juiced. Transfer to a serving glass and add some ice.

Serve immediately.

Nutrition information per serving: Kcal: 272, Protein: 4.8g, Carbs: 79.8g, Fats: 1.7g

33. Pepper Shallot Juice

Ingredients:

1 large bell pepper, seeded

1 small shallot

2 large tomatoes, halved

2 garlic cloves, peeled

3 large cucumbers

1 large lime, peeled

¼ cup of fresh cilantro

Preparation:

Wash the bell pepper and cut into halves. Remove the seeds and chop into small pieces.

Wash the shallots and chop into small pieces set aside.

Wash the tomatoes and place them in a medium bowl. Cut into quarters or small pieces. Reserve the juice while cutting and pour it into serving glasses.

Wash the cucumbers and chop into small pieces. Set aside.

Peel the lime and cut into quarters. Set aside.

Wash the cilantro and roughly chop it. Set aside.

Peel the garlic cloves and set aside.

Process the tomatoes, cucumbers, bell pepper, shallots, lime, garlic, and cilantro.Transfer to serving glasses and refrigerate for 20 minutes before serving.

Nutritional information per serving: Kcal: 109, Protein: 6.4g, Carbs: 38.5g, Fats: 1.2g

34.   Fennel Orange Juice

Ingredients:

1 small fennel

1 large orange, peeled

6 medium-sized radishes

5 large celery stalks

1 large cucumber

Preparation:

Trim off the fennel stalks and wilted outer layers. Wash and cut into bite-sized pieces and set aside.

Peel the orange and divide into wedges.

Wash and cut the radishes into small pieces. Set aside.

Wash the celery and roughly chop into pieces. Set aside.

Wash the cucumber and chop into small pieces. Process all in a juicer, one at a time. Transfer to serving glasses and add some water to adjust the thickness, if needed. Add some ice and serve.

Nutritional information per serving: Kcal: 110, Protein: 6.1g, Carbs: 28.7g, Fats: 1.2g

35.   Celery Apple Juice

Ingredients:

4 celery stalks

1 large green apple, cored

½ cup of green cabbage

3 large carrots

1 large lemon, peeled

1 tbsp of liquid honey

Preparation:

Wash the celery stalks and cut into small chunks. Set aside.

Wash the cabbage and roughly chop it. Set aside.

Peel the lemon and cut into quarters. Set aside.

Wash carrots and celery. Cut into small pieces and place in a medium bowl.

Wash the apple and remove the core. Cut into bite-sized pieces and set aside.

Now, first process the cabbage, then celery, apple, carrots, and lemon. Transfer to serving glasses and stir in the liquid honey.

Add water to adjust the thickness of the juice if you like. However, this is optional.

Refrigerate for about 5 minutes before serving.

Nutritional information per serving: Kcal: 162, Protein: 3.1g, Carbs: 39.3g, Fats: 0.1g

ADDITIONAL TITLES FROM THIS AUTHOR

70 Effective Meal Recipes to Prevent and Solve Being Overweight: Burn Fat Fast by Using Proper Dieting and Smart Nutrition

By

Joe Correa CSN

48 Acne Solving Meal Recipes: The Fast and Natural Path to Fixing Your Acne Problems in Less Than 10 Days!

By

Joe Correa CSN

41 Alzheimer's Preventing Meal Recipes: Reduce or Eliminate Your Alzheimer's Condition in 30 Days or Less!

By

Joe Correa CSN

70 Effective Breast Cancer Meal Recipes: Prevent and Fight Breast Cancer with Smart Nutrition and Powerful Foods

By

Joe Correa CSN

www.ingramcontent.com/pod-product-compliance
Lightning Source LLC
Chambersburg PA
CBHW030244030426
42336CB00009B/241